W9-BHM-938

What Every Woman Must Know About Heart Disease

Also by Siegfried J. Kra

Is Surgery Necessary?

Examine Your Doctor

Aging Myths: Reversible Causes of Mind and Memory Loss

Coronary Bypass Surgery: Who Needs It?

The Three-Legged Stallion and Other Tales from a Doctor's Notebook

Concise Echocardiography

Deductive Echocardiography

Echocardiography Case Book

Textbook of Physical Diagnosis

What Every Woman Must Know About Heart Disease

A No-nonsense Approach to Diagnosing, Treating, and Preventing the #1 Killer of Women

Siegfried J. Kra, M.D., F.A.C.P.

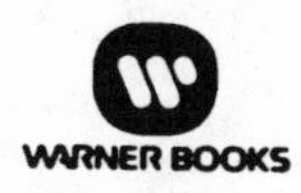

A Time Warner Company

This book is not intended as a substitute for medical advice. The reader should regularly consult a physician or health care professional in matters relating to health and particularly in respect to any symptoms which may require diagnosis or medical attention.

Warner Books, Inc., 1271 Avenue of the Americas, New York, NY 10020

A Time Warner Company

Printed in the United States of America

First Printing: March 1996

10 9 8 7 6 5 4 3 2 1

Library of Congress Cataloging-in-Publication Data

Kra, Siegfried J.

What every woman must know about heart disease : a no-nonsense approach to diagnosing, treating, and preventing the #1 killer of women / Siegfried J. Kra.

p. cm.

Includes index.

ISBN 0-446-51986-3

1. Heart—Diseases—Popular works. 2. Women—Diseases.

I. Title.

RC672.K73 1995 94-24691

616.1'2'0082—dc20 CIP

Book design by Giorgetta Bell McRee

TO LISETTE AND ANNICE

Acknowledgments

I wish to give thanks to the following erudite people who made so many sound suggestions in the preparation of this book:
The Hon. Linda B. Johnson, Commissioner of Workers' Compensation for the state of Connecticut; Gloria Schaeffers, Commissioner of Consumer Affairs for the state of Connecticut; Ann Kern, Vice President of Korn-Ferry, Inc.; Dr. M. Antonia Gotto, Jr., Chairman, Department of Medicine, Baylor College of Medicine, Houston, Texas; Dr. Rennee Langou, Associate Clinical Professor, Yale School of Medicine; Dr. S. Hashim, Associate Clinical Professor of Cardiothoracic Surgery, Yale School of Medicine; Dr. A. Evans, Professor of Epidemiology, Yale School of Medicine; my agent Sue Cohen; my two editors Robin Levenson and Jamie Raab; my two daughters Lisette and Annice Kra; and the endlessly supportive Lita Pridgeon.

Contents

What Every Woman Must Know About Heart Disease

Introduction

For thousands of years, the major cause of premature death among women stemmed directly from pregnancy. As late as the eighteenth century, epidemics of so-called childbirth fever in Paris and Vienna—among the most sophisticated of cities—killed at least one in five women who conceived. Not until the mid-nineteenth century, under the leadership of Dr. Ignaz Semmelweis, were medical students instructed in such rudimentary hygiene as washing their hands before participating in a delivery. It took another twenty years for the medical profession to finally accept Dr. Semmelweis's theory that unsterile hands transmitted infection in the delivery room. Even so, countless people throughout the centuries, and even well into this one, went directly from milking cows to delivering babies without a thought of the inevitable infection that would follow. Today, thankfully, maternal death during childbirth is exceedingly rare in developed nations.

Women now face an entirely different threat to their

lives and well-being: heart disease. By 1950, deaths from heart disease were increasing in women even as they were declining in men. Currently in the United States, a woman's life is more likely to be cut short by a heart attack or stroke than by cancer of the breast or lung. For women over age sixty, heart disease has become the major cause of death. Heart attacks kill 250,000 women each year in the United States—almost half of the 540,000 Americans who die of heart attacks annually. Heart disease accounts for one third of all deaths among American women. Yet, physicians too often overlook the possibility of heart disease in their female patients. Why?

When I first started practicing medicine thirty years ago, every textbook on cardiology described the classic symptoms of heart disease only as they occurred in men. Even later, when cholesterol was identified as one of the culprits responsible for clogging the arteries of the heart, it was widely assumed that this process afflicted men only. I am embarrassed to recall a time when I would routinely tell female patients how lucky they were to be able to enjoy all the steaks and chops they desired without fear of hurting their hearts.

This attitude was based on evidence that men historically comprised the vast majority of fatal heart-attack victims. In fact, being male was considered the major risk factor for developing a heart attack, and being female was assumed to offer virtual immunity from cardiac disease. As life spans increased over the last few generations, however, it became painfully clear that this was no longer the case. Heart disease can now be considered an area in which women have achieved full equality with men.

Nonetheless, the myth of female immunity to heart disease persists. As a result, heart disease in women is often overlooked and misdiagnosed; their physical symptoms are frequently ascribed to the many other conditions that heart disease mimics. Often, women are denied the same diagnostic tests used routinely to evaluate heart disease in men. Even such basic procedures as electrocardiograms and exercise stress tests are used inconsistently on female patients.

These inequities persist even after the Framingham Heart Study—one of the largest and most respected studies of heart disease to date—made clear in 1983 that heart attack is not an overwhelmingly male phenomenon. In fact, heart attack has become the most common cause of death in postmenopausal women. The Framingham Study, issued by the National Heart, Lung and Blood Institute, spurred a plethora of population studies, which confirmed the Framingham findings.

Nonetheless, some researchers still bought into the myth that women develop heart disease much less often than men. For example, the 1987 Coronary Artery Surgical Study (CASS), sponsored by the National Institutes of Health (NIH), included no women over age sixty. Because of this oversight, CASS found that 50 percent of the women with chest pain who underwent an X ray of their coronary arteries (angiography) had normal arteries, while almost 80 percent of men had evidence of blockages. This led CASS researchers to the faulty conclusion that female heart disease was less prevalent and women therefore did not need as many diagnostic tests.

To avoid the kind of bias that skewed the CASS results, the NIH has now mandated that all researchers receiving NIH grants must include a full range of women in their cardiovascular studies.

Our new awareness of heart-disease risks in women was driven home in Heart Association meetings in the past two years. Women and heart disease was one of the major themes of the presentations.

Despite the growing number of heart-disease deaths

among women, there are reasons for optimism. Coronary artery disease is not only a reversible illness, but women can expect to respond to medical treatment as men do. And like men, women can take many steps to protect themselves against heart disease. Because heart disease often manifests differently in females, however, women require prevention and treatment programs tailored to their particular physical needs.

This book will discuss, clearly and comprehensively, the newest information about the causes of heart disease in women, its treatments and preventions. Readers will learn about the latest research findings, including some that have yet to be incorporated into standard textbooks on cardiology used by medical students. Numerous case studies are included in this book, but readers should note that they are composite sketches for the purposes of illustration and to protect the patients' privacy.

It is my sincere hope that the information and guidelines presented in this book will not only help readers prevent heart disease, but also show women with established heart disease what steps they can take to reverse its progress and prolong their lives.

PART I

DIAGNOSING HEART DISEASE IN WOMEN

CHAPTER 1

WHY MORE WOMEN ARE DYING OF HEART DISEASE

There are some inherent biological differences in the way the heart functions in men and women, differences that are only beginning to be discovered or confirmed. These differences cause the standard heart tests, such as the exercise stress test, to sometimes be difficult to interpret in women; this is one of the reasons why women undergo less stress testing than men and receive fewer X rays designed to detect abnormalities in their coronary arteries.

As a consequence, heart disease in women frequently goes undiscovered until it reaches advanced stages—when the likelihood of a woman dying from her first heart attack is much greater. Women also tend to have more serious complications from coronary bypass operations.

Perhaps because their hearts function differently, women may exhibit different symptoms of heart disease than men. Women, for example, tend not to experience classic chest pain during a heart attack; instead, they often experience shortness of breath or fatigue. To make matters worse, many women's first heart attacks can swiftly be followed by a second, which may well be fatal because their arteries seem less able to compensate for the partial death of heart muscle that a heart attack can leave in its wake.

Researchers have been unable to pinpoint why heart disease and heart-related deaths have increased among women. Dr. Nanette Kay Wenger, professor of medicine at Emory University, has summarized what we do know about women and heart disease: Generally, women develop heart-disease symptoms about ten years later than men, and women are usually about twenty years older than men when they suffer their first heart attacks. Estrogen, a female hormone, protects the female heart until about five to ten years following menopause. Women whose ovaries are surgically removed before natural menopause apparently have an eightfold increased risk of suffering a heart attack. Nonsmoking women under age sixty-five still suffer far fewer heart attacks than men.

STRESS AND HEART DISEASE

Over the last three decades, the number of women working outside the home has risen dramatically. Is career-related stress a reason why the heart-attack rate among women has gone up? Let's consider these two case studies.

Beatrice was forty-four years old, married, with two teenage sons. A legal secretary, Beatrice's alarm roused her at six each morning, and she often didn't fall asleep until midnight. Her secretarial job was relentlessly stressful. Once she was home, she had little physical or mental energy left to fulfill her other roles: mothering, keeping house, and being a wife and lover. Her husband, a salesman, typically spent five days a week on the road.

For many years, Beatrice smoked two packs of cigarettes a day, sometimes more, and she took oral contraceptives. Each night before going to bed, she drank a large tumbler of brandy with her final three cigarettes. Only then was she able to fall asleep.

For seven years, Beatrice did her best to earn money and take care of her family, but everything seemed to fall apart when one of her sons was arrested for selling drugs. One night soon afterward, I received a phone call from Beatrice complaining of severe heartburn. Knowing her habits and lifestyle, I suspected something much more serious. I met her in the hospital emergency room. Her electrocardiogram (ECG) revealed that she had just survived a heart attack.

Despite the constant stress she was under, Beatrice's heart attack was not caused by stress alone. Women who smoke have a 40 percent greater chance of suffering a heart attack before menopause compared with nonsmokers. For reasons not yet understood, women smokers who also take birth control pills double their heart-attack risk. (The pill does not increase heart-attack risk in nonsmokers.) The inner walls of Beatrice's coronary arteries were damaged, which allowed cholesterol deposits to form.

Despite her stress, Beatrice probably would have avoided the heart attack if she had exercised regularly, followed a low-fat diet, and didn't smoke. But Beatrice was a heart attack waiting to happen. Learning that her son had been arrested was the apparent trigger. The anxiety that followed raised her blood pressure, increased her pulse, and accelerated the blockage in the already-damaged arteries. If Beatrice had normal arteries, she probably would have weathered the news about her son without suffering a heart attack. But her history of poor health habits had left her vulnerable.

* * *

Lila, fifty, was divorced and living alone. A nonsmoker, Lila worked as a teacher in a "problem" New York City school. Both her parents had heart disease.

When she developed mild high blood pressure (hypertension), Lila asked me to write a letter to her principal requesting that some of her duties be changed since she was under constant stress from her unruly class and from her supervisor, who was harassing her. Lila was convinced that stress on the job precipitated her hypertension. Nonetheless, her principal refused to make the changes we had requested.

Soon thereafter, Lila suffered a heart attack in her classroom. She underwent a cardiac catheterization, a procedure in which a thin, flexible tube is threaded into the coronary arteries to deliver a dye that is visible on a specialized X ray. The test showed that one of her arteries was blocked and that a fresh blood clot had formed, bringing on the heart attack. Lila apparently had a partial blockage in her artery for some time. The pressure of her job, a genetic susceptibility to heart disease, and the onset of hypertension undoubtedly were responsible for the attack. Luckily, Lila recovered and was able to teach again. But this time, she found a job in a different school, one she found less stressful.

There are 52 million working women in the United States, 25 percent of whom are single parents, and many suffer from severe stress. Despite the role stress played in both Beatrice's and Lila's heart attacks, there is no solid evidence to suggest that the increase in the number of working women has raised the overall cardiovascular death rate. According to one expert who spoke at a recent seminar on women's health sponsored by the NIH, the influx of women in the workplace is too recent to form conclusions about whether women under extreme stress are at special risk for a heart attack.

Indeed, numerous studies to date suggest quite the opposite. Stress in an otherwise healthy person does not make her more prone to a heart attack. The so-called type A personality—characterized as an individual who is aggressive, compulsive, and generally frantic—does not seem more likely to suffer a heart attack than the woman who is just the opposite—the calm, type B personality.

CHAPTER 2

UNDERSTANDING SYMPTOMS OF HEART DISEASE IN WOMEN

When we think "heart attack," we usually envision a man clutching at his chest, his face twisted with pain and terror. This is a typical male reaction to an attack of angina, which is derived from the Greek for "strangulation."

Angina is a signal that the heart is not receiving an adequate supply of oxygen. The cause is usually a blockage in the arteries feeding the heart. The pain, similar to a cramp in the leg after running, arises because the muscle—the heart—is not receiving enough blood and is starved for oxygen.

For the most part, chest pain in women, particularly in young women, is not due to heart disease. It usually stems from any of several conditions described later in this chapter. When women do have heart attacks, they may not suffer the angina that is so typical among males. That is, all the symptoms of their coronary artery disease may masquerade as another illness, such as mitral valve prolapse syndrome (see Chapter 6) or acid indigestion.

As pointed out in Chapter 1, women have been excluded from most studies on coronary artery disease until recently. As a result, relatively little is known about heart-disease symptoms in women. As numerous clinical studies have shown, doctors use male symptoms as a standard and are therefore less likely to recognize heart disease in women.

Even when a female patient does exhibit the classic male symptoms, doctors still typically overlook the possibility of heart disease. Indeed, some women have actually died of a heart attack simply because they are women; their symptoms were dismissed or misdiagnosed because of their gender. Believe it or not, many heart-attack victims (both men and women) were examined by a physician within two weeks prior to the attack, but their problem went undetected.

Take, for example, the case of Mildred, a fifty-two-year-old woman who awoke early one morning with a toothache. She visited her dentist, who dutifully took X rays of her teeth. He said she needed nothing more than a good cleaning.

When the pain in her tooth worsened, Mildred's dentist referred her to an orthodontist. He suspected temporomandibular joint syndrome (TMJ), also known as teeth-grinding. Mildred was given an uncomfortable mouth brace to wear at night. When the pain spread to her jaw, she consulted an oral surgeon, who told her, "If it doesn't improve, we will have to break your jaw and reset it."

Mildred's jaw pain grew excruciating. She went to the emergency room of her local hospital where she was examined by an eminent cardiologist. Her electrocardiogram results were normal, so the doctor sent her home. She died of a heart attack in her bed three hours later.

Jaw pain is a common symptom of heart disease. If Mildred had been a man, she probably would have been admitted to the hospital for observation in spite of the normal electrocardiogram. If a heart attack is in its early stages, it may take hours or even days to show up on the ECG.

Today we realize that all symptoms—chest pain and other types of symptoms—must be thoroughly investigated regardless of the patient's gender. This is particularly true in female patients who have heart-disease risk factors, such as smoking, smoking in combination with taking birth control pills, high cholesterol, diabetes, or who are postmenopausal.

How, then, do women experience heart disease? As we have seen, the classic male symptoms of heart disease are frequently absent in women, and the cardiac symptoms women commonly suffer can mimic other medical problems. Patients and physicians alike should be aware of the following potential symptoms of heart disease in women:

BACK PAIN. Back pain in both men and women can arise from a myriad of causes, including muscle strain or spasm, osteoporosis (thinning bones that fracture easily), a degenerative disc, trauma, a tumor of the spine, an ulcer, cancer of the pancreas, or coronary artery disease. In women, back pain is commonly attributed to depression, especially if the woman has had a hysterectomy. (Depression is very common after a hysterectomy.)

Women tend to report psychosomatic symptoms more often than men, and physicians frequently will regard a female patient's complaint of upper back pain as a psychosomatic symptom of depression. By contrast, a man complaining of severe back pain will routinely be given an ECG and a chest X ray to try to ascertain whether he is suffering a heart attack or has a ruptured blood vessel.

As women become older, the chances increase that the cause of high back pain is not depression, but may be coronary artery disease. The right coronary artery feeds the back of the heart (the inferior wall). If stimulated, nerves from that area can shoot pain to the upper and lower back. One of the common symptoms of an inferior wall heart attack is back pain. It is incumbent upon the doctor to investigate all potential causes of a female patient's back pain—including the possibility of heart disease.

FATIGUE. Tiring easily is a common symptom of heart disease in both women and men. The patient may complain about losing energy over a period of weeks, thinking he or she was coming down with the flu. Then suddenly, the patient is hit with chest pain as though struck by a cannonball.

Fatigue stemming from heart disease results from the weakened heart pumping out insufficient amounts of blood, which causes low blood pressure. In the male patient, fatigue more often than not is viewed as a sign that something is seriously wrong, especially if its onset is new. When it comes to a woman's fatigue, however, most doctors disregard it rather than investigating whether heart disease is a potential cause. They believe that women simply are more likely to complain of loss of energy. To be sure, fatigue is a common symptom of depression, but it also can be the first clue of heart disease.

SWEATING. Caused by an outpouring of adrenaline, sweating may accompany angina or a heart attack. During a heart attack, the heart loses its power to contract because its blood supply is shut off. The falling blood pressure triggers the body's internal pharmacy to secrete adrenaline, which acts to raise the blood pressure, increase the pulse, and make the arteries dilate. All this causes sweat to seep out of the pores of the skin.

Sweating is more likely to be reported by men than by women, whose sweat glands do not evacuate as easily. "Doc," a male patient may say, "the pain started like a tiger ripping my chest open, and I became drenched with sweat. It was like I just climbed out of the shower, but I always sweat a lot anyway."

Women tend to sweat less and also may be less descriptive about their symptoms. When I asked one very proper female patient whether she experienced any perspiration with her chest pain, she replied, "Well, I did become a little overheated."

FAINTING. Fainting, light-headedness, and falling to the ground are symptoms of heart disease and are as common in men as they are in women. The difference lies in other people's reaction to these symptoms.

A middle-aged man who suddenly collapses will be rushed to the hospital to determine the cause. He usually will be admitted for an overnight stay to rule out the possibility of a heart attack. By contrast, a fainting woman will probably be helped to a seat and given a glass of water. A woman who is postmenopausal, who smokes, and who has other coronary risk factors such as diabetes or hypertension should certainly be admitted into the hospital if she faints. The story of Agnes illustrates the importance of fully investigating a fainting spell.

Agnes was a high-strung, successful executive who prided herself on her excellent health. She maintained a low-fat diet and exercised daily. She drank only the occasional glass of wine and never smoked. Her systolic blood pressure, the upper number in a blood pressure reading, rarely rose above 110 (well below 145 to 160, which would indicate borderline or mild hypertension), and her blood cholesterol level was very low.

But Agnes never told anyone that she would become light-headed when rising suddenly from a chair. She interpreted the light-headedness she experienced after her third mile of jogging as a "runner's high."

One evening at a cocktail party, Agnes passed out after drinking a glass of wine. Seconds later, she revived and the following day made a point of seeing her doctor. Her examination proved normal, and the doctor advised her not to drink wine anymore.

But Agnes continued to experience light-headedness. She collapsed one night on her way to the bathroom after a very active sexual experience. The doctor in the emergency room said, "Perhaps there was a bit too much excitement tonight. That can happen, you know."

The doctor on call that evening happened to be a cardiologist, who, as he listened to her heart, heard something strange when Agnes moved from a reclining to a sitting position. Through his stethoscope, the doctor detected a sound like something moving in her chest—not a murmur, but a plopping sound he had never heard before. The next day, he ordered an echocardiogram, a sonar examination of the heart, which confirmed his suspicion: Agnes's heart had a tumor on it, which bounced like a Ping-Pong ball. When Agnes stood up, the tumor blocked the passage of blood from her heart, causing the light-headedness and fainting spells.

Tumors of the heart are rare, but fainting is not and should never be ignored. Fainting may stem from many causes other than a heart attack, including a sudden, irregular, or rapid heartbeat (an arrhythmia) or a sudden drop in blood pressure, both of which result in too little blood reaching the brain. In addition to coronary artery disease, other cardiac and noncardiac conditions also can account for fainting. These include bleeding, dehydration, stroke, fever, and blood poisoning (septicemia).

PALPITATIONS. One of the most common reasons female patients consult a cardiologist is because they have fast or irregular heartbeats. Some patients call them palpitations or skipped beats; some say, "My heart feels like it is going to jump out of my chest."

Irregular or speeding heartbeats are an annoying and frightening symptom. They may cause the patient to feel faint and light-headed and can make the most even-tempered person feel anxious. This understandable reaction establishes a vicious cycle: Fear causes more adrenaline to rush out, which, in turn, increases the heart rate.

There are many possible reasons for palpitations, and the symptom requires a thorough investigation. Coronary artery disease is usually not the cause, but palpitations can be the first sign of a heart attack or a diseased heart valve (see Chapter 7).

SHORTNESS OF BREATH. Another possible early sign of heart disease is shortness of breath. It is a symptom many people ignore for a very long time—until it becomes intolerable. Diabetic women can suffer heart attacks without ever complaining of chest pain. The only sign might be the unexpected onset of weakness, feeling faint, or becoming short of breath.

When asked by a doctor whether she ever becomes short of breath, the patient may say, "I am always short of breath when I climb stairs and when I vacuum." A careful medical history will reveal whether her shortness of breath has become more frequent. I cannot count the times I have asked women in the coronary care unit if they have been more short of breath recently and was told, "Now that you mention it . . ."

Smoking can worsen shortness of breath. According to a recent government survey, more women than men now smoke cigarettes. Smoking-related shortness of breath can stem from chronic bronchitis or emphysema. People with these diseases can find themselves gasping for air merely by walking a few hundred feet.

In heart disease, the weakened heart is no longer able to pump out all the blood from its chambers. This allows fluid to back up into the lungs, causing shortness of breath.

ARTHRITIS AND JOINT PAIN. Arthritis, osteoporosis, and joint pain are very common in postmenopausal women. Arthritis and osteoporosis are not generally life-threatening. Pain produced by these conditions, however, may mask heart disease, which can cause similar pain.

The nerves of the heart that send out pain messages are like a spider's web. At the core of the web is the heart, and its tendrils of pain can radiate in all directions, settling in the face, the jaw, the shoulder, the chest, the arms, the elbow, the neck, the back, and as far down as the navel.

Several years ago, in the middle of the summer, Sally, a patient in her mid-sixties, called my office to complain that her arthritis was acting up in the intense humidity. The worst of it was in her shoulders. "They're killing me," she said. I should have taken her at her word.

I examined her carefully when she came into my office later that day. Sally did have pain when I moved her shoulders, but I could not reproduce the severe pain that brought her to the office.

Sally was a heavy smoker and had a cancerous lung removed a few years earlier. Her ECG results were normal, so I referred her back to her cancer surgeon to explore the possibility of a malignancy in her shoulders. None was found.

The night after she consulted her surgeon, Sally went into cardiac arrest. Her daughter, a nurse, resuscitated her. In the hospital, we swiftly unplugged Sally's blocked coronary arteries with a balloon, a procedure called angioplasty. Her life was saved.

BLOATING. Abdominal bloating is another common complaint among women. Many women know that menstruation is on the way when they feel bloated. But bloating may also be an early sign of coronary artery blockage. Bloating results when the intestine does not receive enough blood. Gas forms because of improper transit and digestion of food.

Carrie, a heavyset woman who became a patient of mine at age forty-four, said that she felt bloated almost every day of her life. But she had so many other medical problems, none of her previous doctors ever suspected heart disease.

Carrie had hypertension, which was easily controlled by medication; high cholesterol; and back trouble. She was unable to lose weight.

The first thing we discovered was that Carrie had stones in her gallbladder. Surgeons removed the diseased organ, which contained twenty small cholesterol stones. Yet, Carrie still felt bloated.

The most dramatic bloating episode occurred when she joined an aerobic dance class. After ten minutes of exercise, she became so bloated that she had to stop; her stomach protruded as though she were pregnant. Her resting electrocardiogram was normal, but she complained of feeling bloated during a cardiac stress test. At this point, her ECG tracing became abnormal, showing characteristics of coronary artery disease.

Further tests revealed that all of the blood vessels in Carrie's heart were critically blocked. After bypass surgery, she felt like a new person.

HEARTBURN, BELCHING, AND OTHER PAIN. Heartburn, belching, and bloating are often initial signs of heart attack for both men and women. But these symptoms may have another source. There is a small recess in the intestine, located on the left side, just under the left breast, called the splenic flexure. It is a miserable little cul-de-sac, a pocket that can trap gas formed by the intestine or swallowed air.

It makes its presence known by pain—chest pain, pain under the left breast, pain that travels down the left arm. Sometimes the pain lasts for hours and is accompanied by sweating and a fast heartbeat; sometimes it can be a stabbing, knifelike pain. A good burp may bring relief. But the pain may not come from the intestine. It may be a sign of coronary disease.

These antics by the splenic flexure can lead a doctor down the wrong path, especially if the ECG is normal. The splenic flexure is likely to be blamed for the discomfort. If the patient is a woman who is overweight and always gassy, the diagnosis of coronary artery disease might well be overlooked.

Another symptom that sometimes masquerades as a different disease is pain on the right side, where the gallbladder is located. This may not indicate gallbladder trouble, however; it can be a sign of a heart attack.

Each episode of these symptoms does not mean that a woman has a heart ailment, but heart disease should be considered a possibility if she is postmenopausal, smokes, and has a strong family history of heart attacks.

CHEST PAIN AND SYNDROME X. Chest pain in a young woman rarely arises from the heart, but it can happen. Therefore all chest pains must be investigated, regardless of the patient's age or gender. Unfortunately, if a young woman has complained of chest pain over the years, and then, postmenopausally, complains to the same doctor of chest pain, it is entirely possible that the physician, conditioned to the complaint, may miss the heart disease.

When women do experience chest pain from heart disease, they usually complain of a heaviness between the breasts, a "sinking feeling," a weakness, or a burning sensation—not the stabbing, seizing pain that men often report. Some describe the feeling as a severe tightness that stops their breath, or as a pain that travels down the left arm to the wrist, or even up to the jaw. The female patient may leave her hand on her chest, as if for relief. Many, though, will describe their pain as men do: "It feels like an elephant sitting on my chest."

I was recently asked to consult on a case of a sturdy forty-four-year-old policewoman. She felt chest pain whenever she chased a suspect. Her beat was a high-crime, drug-ridden area of a medium-sized city. She was a smoker, and her father had died of heart disease. Her married life was excellent, and she enjoyed her work in spite of its dangers and frustrations.

Her ECG was normal, as were her physical examination and her exercise stress test. Her symptoms were nonetheless so suggestive of coronary disease that we performed a thallium stress test (see Chapter 5). The results of the thallium test pointed to blocked coronary arteries. X rays of the arteries through cardiac catheterization were normal, however. We next took X rays of the policewoman's entire gastrointestinal tract, which showed no abnormalities.

Cardiologists often face this dilemma—symptoms with no apparent cause—when trying to diagnose female patients, and sometimes male patients as well. Because we do not understand the cause of this rather common disorder, we call it Syndrome X.

Syndrome X is used to describe women and men who have classical angina pains but normal coronary arteries. In 1892, Sir William Osler, considered the father of modern medicine, taught that angina pains without coronary artery disease were more common in women than in men. These women tend to have associated symptoms of hot flushes, shortness of breath, migraine headaches, and cold hands. Dr. Philip Sarrel, of the Yale School of Medicine, reported in 1992 that many of these women are estrogen deficient, either from surgical removal of their ovaries or natural menopause. Estrogen-replacement therapy resulted in a dramatic improvement in their symptoms.

Chest pain also can sometimes be the result of a condition called Prinzmetal's angina. In this case, the arteries are not blocked, but they twitch or spasm. The condition is more common in women than in men and can be effectively treated with medication.

Chest pain occurring either at rest or during physical exertion also may be a manifestation of mitral valve prolapse syndrome (see Chapter 6).

PERICARDITIS. Pericarditis is an infection of the pericardium, the sac covering the heart. Pericarditis can cause severe chest pain and may be confused with a heart attack. It can occur at any age and is usually caused by a virus.

In most cases, pericarditis pain is worsened when the patient is lying flat and is relieved when he or she is leaning forward. It is sometimes accompanied by difficulty swallowing if the esophagus, which touches the pericardium, also becomes inflamed.

Anti-inflammatory medications give the patient dramatic relief from symptoms. Once in a while, however, pericarditis is caused by blood or tumor cells and becomes a much more serious condition.

When a patient complains of chest pain, it is important to rule out the possibility of pericarditis because if the patient receives clot-dissolving medication (thrombolysis) for an assumed heart attack, dangerous hemorrhages can occur into the inflamed pericardium. The pericardium then must be drained to release the blood or the blood can choke the heart, causing it to fail. Sometimes patients suffer a second episode of chest pain a week or so after a heart attack, the pain being caused by pericarditis.

PNEUMOTHORAX. Many women work out with weights and are very involved in strenuous exercises. I saw one young woman with chest pain after she finished an hour of vigorous isometric (weight-lifting) exercise at her gym. She had difficulty breathing and suffered chest pain each time she took a breath. An X ray showed she had collapsed her lung, a condition known as a pneumothorax.

After a tube was inserted into her chest, the lung expanded and her chest pain disappeared. Against my better judgment, she insisted on resuming her strenuous exercise regime. I expect another emergency call from her any day now because her lung surely will collapse again. This young woman has an inherent weakness of her lung that probably resulted from weight lifting, which causes the pressure inside the chest to rise.

DISSECTING ANEURYSM. The large artery, called the aorta, that arises from the heart like a stem of the amaryllis flower, can enlarge and split down the center. This is a life-threatening condition called a dissecting aneurysm. It causes severe chest pain.

The doctor will suspect this condition if the pain is extremely severe but the ECG is normal. It can be definitively diagnosed with a CAT scan or arteriogram (an X ray of the aorta). Surgery can repair the dissecting aneurysm in some cases, but a delay in diagnosis usually causes death.

When a woman experiences any of the symptoms described in this chapter, it certainly does not mean that she has a heart ailment. It does mean, however, that the possibility of heart disease exists and should be thoroughly explored by a physician. This is especially important for women who are postmenopausal, smoke, or have a family history of heart disease.

CHAPTER 3

CORONARY RISK FACTORS IN WOMEN (AND HOW THEY DIFFER FROM MEN'S)

There are a variety of risk factors involved in female heart disease. Some, such as heredity, cannot be avoided. But as you will see in this chapter, most risk factors—smoking, being overweight, not getting enough exercise, eating fatty foods—can be eliminated if you have the willpower. Through education, I believe that women will find the motivation to take better care of their hearts and overall health. If enough women follow the advice laid out in this chapter and teach their daughters to do the same, I predict that, in future generations, female heart disease will become a rare entity indeed.

CHOLESTEROL AND THE FEMALE HEART

By now, almost everybody has heard of cholesterol, and many people even know their blood cholesterol level. Cholesterol screenings have become almost as common as blood pressure screenings in supermarkets, shopping malls, and health fairs around the United States. You may think you're fine if your cholesterol number is under 200 or in trouble if your number is greater than that. But the information provided by most cholesterol screenings is far too general to provide meaningful information about your health. Let's examine cholesterol and other blood fats in more detail.

Cholesterol is a fat found in animal foods and dairy products. Three quarters of this yellow, greasy substance is manufactured by the human liver, and the remainder comes from what we eat. Despite its bad reputation, cholesterol is an essential component of life. It is needed to make estrogen, vitamins, and the coverings of all the nerves. Unfortunately, excessive amounts of a certain form of cholesterol is the major cause of atherosclerosis (hardening of the arteries characterized by deposits of cholesterol plaques) and coronary artery disease.

Like all fats, cholesterol floats in water, and blood is mostly water. Blood also contains proteins called lipoproteins. The type of lipoprotein that binds to cholesterol and carries it to all the arteries is called low-density lipoprotein, or LDL. The cholesterol plaque found in clogged coronary arteries is made up mostly of LDL. This is why LDL is sometimes called the "bad cholesterol."

The so-called "good cholesterol"—high-density lipoprotein, or HDL—carries the cholesterol away from the walls of the arteries and back to the liver.

Another type of blood fat derived from dietary fat and sugars is called triglyceride. When a doctor orders a blood test known as a lipid profile, the laboratory measures all kinds of blood fats: cholesterol, triglycerides, LDL, and HDL. Lipid profile results are most accurate when the test is performed after you have fasted for ten to twelve hours. For most people, having blood drawn for the test early in the morning, before eating breakfast, is most convenient.

The National Institutes of Health has issued these guidelines for both men and women:

- Cholesterol less than 180 milligrams (mg) is desirable.
- Cholesterol of 200–239 mg is borderline to high risk for heart disease.
- Cholesterol greater than 240 mg is high risk.
- HDL greater than 40 mg is desirable.
- LDL less than 120 mg is desirable.
- LDL more than 160 mg is high risk.

It is not enough just to measure the cholesterol levels. All the lipids, or blood fats, must be known in order to determine your risks for a heart attack and stroke. Here are some more guidelines:

- Triglycerides less than 200 mg is desirable.
- The higher the HDL, the lower the risk for a heart attack.
- The higher the LDL, the greater the risk for a heart attack.
- A good number for the HDL is above 50.
- An HDL level of 30 is considered dangerous.

Until they pass through menopause, women have much higher levels of cholesterol and HDL than men. The HDL offers a degree of protection against atherosclerosis. After menopause, a woman's cholesterol may remain elevated, but the HDL level drops. For women, the overall cholesterol count is not as revealing as the levels of LDL, HDL, and triglycerides. Many elderly women, for example, have cholesterol levels above 260 but are free of coronary artery disease because their HDL is above 50 and their triglyceride level is normal.

Premenopausal women at greatest risk for a heart attack have a cholesterol count above 240, an HDL below 35, an LDL above 200, and a triglyceride level above 400 mg. Most nonsmoking women of childbearing age have HDL levels above 50. Smoking lowers the HDL dramatically. Postmenopausal women who don't smoke are not considered at serious risk for a heart attack if their cholesterol reading is above 250 and their HDL is over 60.

Postmenopausal women with cholesterol levels above 260, LDL above 200, and an HDL below 35 are considered at risk, especially if they smoke.

Elevated triglycerides (above 250 mg) is regarded as a much greater risk factor for coronary artery disease in women than it is in men. But most patients, male and female, concern themselves with the cholesterol number only.

"My cholesterol is only 200," one woman complained to me from the coronary care unit. "How can I be having a heart attack?"

The reason was obvious to me. Her HDL was 30, her LDL was 200, and she smoked heavily.

At the opposite end of the spectrum was an eighty-five-year-old patient who begged me to put her on cholesterol-lowering medication. "My cholesterol is 290. Why don't you do something?" she said. "Don't I need a diet and pills?

"After all," she continued, "all my friends tell me my cholesterol count is dangerously high. They are on pills."

Despite her advanced age, this woman swam two miles a day. Her HDL was a stellar 90 and her LDL was a normal 120.

Very often, I cannot convince patients that they are in good shape, and they shop around until they find a doctor who gives them medication. It certainly is better to have a low cholesterol count, especially if you can achieve it with diet alone. But, as you can see, this is not by any means the whole story.

Until a few years ago when the medical community

began to seriously look at the HDL and LDL measurements, it was difficult to explain why so many patients with "normal" cholesterol counts still suffered heart attacks. Now it is easier to understand. Another way to predict who is at risk is to look at the ratios of one kind of lipid to another. The LDL-to-HDL ratio should be around 3 to 1; the cholesterol-to-HDL ratio should not be greater than 6 to 1.

WHO SHOULD BE TESTED? Every woman should have her lipid profile performed at least once. This profile must include cholesterol, HDL, LDL, and triglycerides. It is important that a solid, reliable laboratory be used, and that you fast for ten to twelve hours prior to the test. If there are major abnormalities, such as a very low HDL or a very high overall cholesterol count, it is good practice to repeat the test at different times, using different laboratories.

The HDL can be very low in both men and women who smoke. Indeed, the most obvious medical markers of smoking are low HDL and a decrease in lung function. The lower the HDL, the higher the risk for a heart attack. HDL can also be lowered by some otherwise beneficial drugs. Ironically, some of the very drugs used to treat hypertension and angina can lower the HDL. Among them are diuretics and beta-blockers.

Exercise, quitting smoking, and drinking two to four ounces of alcohol daily raise the HDL. Some studies have shown that one or two drinks a day can raise the HDL level by 10 to 15 percent. Giving up smoking can raise an HDL of 30 mg to 40 mg or more. Taking estrogen-replacement therapy after menopause also raises the HDL.

Each rise of 1 mg of HDL reduces the risk for coronary artery disease by 3 percent.

WHERE DOES DIETARY CHOLESTEROL COME FROM? Saturated fats are the major sources of cholesterol, and specific foods such as egg yolks, sweetbreads, and liver are the main sources. Saturated fats are also found in ice cream, butter, whole milk, soft cheeses, beef, poultry, lard, and coconut, palm, and other tropical oils. These fats raise the level of bad cholesterol in the blood and interfere with the removal of cholesterol from the walls of the arteries.

Unsaturated fats do not contribute to cholesterol. They help to lower the cholesterol in the blood by lowering the LDL. Unsaturated fats, also called polyunsaturated fats, are found in such liquid oils as cottonseed, safflower, soybean, and corn. Unsaturated fats also are found in pecans and almonds.

Another type of beneficial fat is found primarily in seafood. Some studies have shown that eating fish more than twice a week reduces heart disease by 50 percent over a twenty-year period. Researchers came to these conclusions by observing the Eskimos, the Japanese, and the inhabitants of Zutphen, Holland, all of whom eat tremendous amounts of fish.

Shellfish had a bad reputation because it was thought to be high in cholesterol. Recent studies, however, have found clams, oysters, and scallops to be low in bad cholesterol. Shrimp and lobster, which had the worst reputations of all, actually have an insignificant impact on a person's cholesterol level. Indeed, a 1982 study disclosed that eating shellfish has no effect on a person's blood cholesterol whatsoever.

The reason seafood is so beneficial may be because of its Omega-3 fatty acid, which helps prevent the clotting of blood (platelet aggregation), and may help prevent atherosclerosis. Salmon, sardines, mackerel, herring, bluefish, and halibut are rich in Omega-3 acid. It is unknown whether taking fish oil in capsule form is beneficial. Fish oil supplements are not regulated by the U.S. Food and Drug Administration, and their long-term effects have not been established. The American Heart Association does not recommend taking supplements of fish oil. Fish oil has been reported to increase bleeding tendencies and decrease the immune system.

The most healthful form of fat is monosaturated fat, which is found in such foods as olive oil, peanuts, avocados, canola oil, and cashews. Monosaturated fat seems to be better than polyunsaturated fat for raising the HDL and lowering the LDL.

Compared with the United States, low death rates from heart disease have consistently been reported in Spain, Italy, Greece, and France. Experts suspect this may stem in part from the heavy use of olive oil and the drinking of red wine in those countries.

SMOKING

Smoking is the major cause of heart attacks and strokes in women. In addition, cigarettes are a major contributing cause of coronary artery and vascular diseases, peptic ulcers, and cancer of the lungs, throat, and bladder, in both sexes. Cigarettes kill more Americans each year than the total number of Americans killed in World War II, the Korean conflict, and the Vietnam War combined. In my experience, almost every premenopausal woman who has suffered a heart attack was a smoker.

In the United States, 30 percent of women smoke cigarettes, and the numbers are not decreasing, nor is women's death rate from heart disease and lung cancer. In fact, in addition to there being more female smokers than male, the number of young female smokers has surpassed the number of young male smokers in recent years.

Nicotine, a powerful poison, is the most addictive component of cigarette smoke. The average American cigarette contains 10 mg of nicotine. Once inhaled by the lungs, nicotine travels to the brain, heart, and eventually reaches all the blood vessels of the body, including the coronary arteries. When we injected nicotine into rats in medical school, it caused instant death. Nicotine is far from the only toxin in cigarettes. Other poisons released in smoke include nitrogen oxides, carbon monoxide, ammonia, nitrosamines, and aromatic amines. Carbon monoxide aggravates coronary artery disease, and the amines cause cancer.

Cigarettes cause the heart to beat faster and constrict the blood vessels, making the heart work harder than it normally would. Smoking also makes the blood clot faster and reduces the amount of oxygen in the bloodstream. Any health benefit achieved from exercise is negated by smoking; exercise can actually be dangerous to smokers. A smoker who exercises strenuously makes her heart work harder and demand more oxygen, which her body cannot supply. A heart attack or a stroke can result because most long-term smokers have already developed atherosclerosis.

Female smokers who suffer from angina generally respond poorly to angina medications. They also tend to have worse outcomes than nonsmokers after coronary bypass surgery. Women with poor circulation of the legs who have pain in their calves when walking will intensify the pain if they continue to smoke. Diabetic women who smoke are more prone to coronary artery disease.

Smoking accelerates hardening of the arteries and is one of the main reasons clots form in the arteries of the legs and brain. Cigarettes also cause a reduction in the level of HDL—the good cholesterol that protects the coronary arteries.

With cigarettes having so many detrimental effects, why do women continue to smoke in increasing numbers? Here are some of the most common reasons I have heard during my years of practice:

"I will gain twenty pounds in a month if I quit."

"You have to die of something."

"It relaxes me." (How can it if it increases the heart rate and constricts the blood vessels?)

"I know it's a bad habit. I just can't help it."

It is very difficult to persuade most women to give up cigarettes—that is, until they land in the coronary care unit. Then some quit, but not all. Some women who have had a lung removed, and even some who have had a heart transplant, return to smoking when they are able to breathe more freely again. But they will probably not get a second chance.

Male smokers are somewhat less difficult to convince to give up the habit, probably because gaining weight is less of a consideration for them.

If a woman were to stop smoking today, her elevated risk of a heart attack would disappear in as little as three years; it takes five years for a man. Quitting smoking slows, and may even halt, the rapid progression of hardening of the arteries. The risk of having a stroke also would decline soon after the last puff.

ORAL CONTRACEPTIVES AND SMOKING. When combined with smoking, oral contraceptives, especially those with high levels of estrogen, are associated with a 40 percent increased heart-attack risk. The reason for this is speculative.

When taken by nonsmokers, the newer birth control pills seem to have no impact on either LDL or HDL and do not advance hardening of the arteries. Some of the older contraceptive pills contained more estrogens and progesterone and produced a slight rise in the LDL and a decrease in the HDL.

Estrogen in birth control pills can elevate a woman's blood pressure. This occurs because estrogens increase sodium retention, which can cause weight gain, bloating, and swelling of the ankles. Some women are more susceptible to these negative effects than others.

If you are a nonsmoker and have normal blood pressure, birth control pills should not raise your risk for a heart attack.

COCAINE

One of the major causes of sudden death in young women and men is abuse of illicit drugs, especially cocaine. According to U.S. government estimates, some 30 million men and women have tried cocaine, and 6 million are regular users. Cocaine use is so widespread that any young person who is having a heart attack or an irregular heartbeat in the emergency room at Yale New Haven Hospital is tested for drug abuse.

Sudden death is not always dose-related, and it is not at all predictable. Cocaine can cause the blood pressure to rise, the heart rate to increase, and the arteries to spasm and become constricted, as though they were packed with cholesterol. Cocaine can cause strokes, heart failure, heart attacks, and blood clots in the lungs.

So many Americans have early coronary artery disease that it is surprising to me that the number of people who die each year from cocaine abuse is not higher.

DIABETES

Diabetes is a cruel, incurable disease in which the pancreas fails to produce enough insulin, a hormone that enables cells to absorb sugar needed for energy. Diabetes affects about 5 million people in the United States, and there are probably another 5 million walking around with undiagnosed diabetes.

Type II diabetes, or adult-onset diabetes, usually surfaces around age forty. Ninety-five percent of women with adult-onset diabetes are obese. These patients are usually treated with dietary changes and oral agents and don't generally need to take insulin to control their blood sugar level. Insulin is taken by type I diabetics, those who developed the illness earlier in life.

For unknown reasons, women diabetics, who outnumber male diabetics, tend to die at a younger age.

Diabetes can affect different systems throughout the body, including the circulatory system, the nervous system, and the cardiovascular system. It is diagnosed when the blood sugar level rises above the normal 130 mg, poisoning all the cells of the body.

Diabetics are more likely than the average person to have high blood pressure, and diabetes increases the heart-attack risk in women fourfold. Diabetes also causes a rise in the cholesterol and triglyceride levels.

Not all women with diabetes develop heart disease, however. In fact, some severely diabetic women I have cared for have hypertension, obesity, and eye and kidney problems, but for some reason some do not have coronary artery disease.

Diabetic women who do develop heart problems seem to have dulled pain sensations and may not realize it when they are stricken with a heart attack. Their main complaints focus on shortness of breath and fatigue, or palpitations.

If you have a family history of diabetes you should have your blood sugar level checked at least once a year. Also report to your doctor any of the early warning signs of diabetes: increased thirst, frequent urination, and fatigue.

Exercise and weight reduction, with strict fat and sugar restrictions, can lessen, and perhaps prevent, the onset of this dreadful illness. Smoking does not seem to trigger diabetes, but there is no question that it complicates active diabetes, possibly to a fatal degree.

OBESITY

Dr. William Osler once said, "When I see a fat person coming in the front door, I want to leave by the back door." His words echo the frustration felt by many physicians when they try to get their obese patients to lose weight. Many doctors say it can be easier to perform a heart transplant or brain surgery.

When a person is 20 to 30 percent over ideal weight, he or she is considered obese. Another way of identifying obesity is by measurements. A woman whose waist measures more than 80 percent of her hips is much more likely to suffer a heart attack than a woman of normal weight. These so-called apple-shaped women are also at greater risk for diabetes, hypertension, stroke, and cancer. Cholesterol from a fat belly enters into the bloodstream more freely than from the hips.

According to an eight-year study from Brigham and Women's Hospital, being just slightly overweight also increases one's heart-attack risk. A women who is 20 percent over her ideal weight increases her chance of having a heart attack by 30 percent, and obese women sustain more heart attacks than obese men.

MENOPAUSE

The biological changes leading to menopause usually begin by the middle or late forties. Some women enter menopause earlier, and others later. As women age, the body gradually decreases its production of estrogen. As menopause begins, periods often become irregular before they finally cease. The myriad of symptoms, such as hot flashes, depression, bloating, a general feeling of malaise, and vaginal dryness, may begin years before menopause and continue for a long time afterward without estrogen-replacement therapy.

As noted earlier, heart disease among premenopausal women is relatively rare. In fact, heart disease kills four men for every woman until the onset of menopause. By age sixty, as women's estrogen level dwindles, their death rate from heart attacks begins to equal or surpass that of men.

Why do women become more vulnerable to heart disease after menopause? Among other things, estrogen is responsible for keeping the level of HDL—the good cholesterol—high, and LDL—the bad cholesterol—in the low range. As women grow older, their estrogen level drops, and so does the protective HDL. At the same time, the LDL rises.

Another important role of estrogen is to keep the blood vessels from constricting and reducing the flow of blood to the heart. If blood vessels constrict, chest pain and heart attacks can occur.

Another group of hormonelike substances, called prostaglandins, also offer some protection against heart disease. Secreted by the premenopausal uterus, prostaglandins dilate the arteries and help prevent blood from clotting.

Beginning estrogen-replacement therapy as soon as menopause (natural or as a result of removal of both ovaries) starts, or even later in the postmenopausal period, has been shown to lower a woman's heart-disease risk substantially. But estrogen-replacement therapy has been associated in many studies with an increased risk of breast and uterine cancers. It's important to discuss the relative risks and benefits of estrogen replacement with your doctor before deciding if it's for you.

HIGH BLOOD PRESSURE (HYPERTENSION)

Centuries ago, measurements of blood pressure were first made by inserting a glass tube into a horse's artery and observing the column of blood surge upward. Modern blood pressure devices employ a column of mercury that is linked to a hollow cuff, which goes around the arm. The cuff is filled with air until blood flow stops. As air is slowly released from the cuff, circulation in the arm returns and the mercury level indicates how much pressure is in the blood vessels when the heart contracts and between each contraction. It is these two readings that define the blood pressure.

The upper number, called systolic pressure, represents the force of blood exerted against the arterial wall. The lower number, called diastolic pressure, represents the relaxation of the blood vessels and heart. It is during the diastolic relaxation that the coronary arteries receive the flow of blood to nourish the heart muscle. Normal blood pressure is about 120/70 for adults of both sexes. If the systolic reading is above 135 and the diastolic reading is 90 or greater on two or three different days, the person is diagnosed as being early hypertensive.

Overall, women have much lower blood pressure than men until they reach about fifty-five years of age. After that, average blood pressure is about the same for women and men. Most of the estimated 60 million Americans with hypertension are fifty-five or older. And fully half of African-Americans have hypertension. High blood

New Classification of Hypertension

Category	Systolic (mmHg)	Diastolic (mmHg)
Normal	<130	<85
High normal	130–139	85–89
Hypertension Stage 1 (Mild)	140–159	90–99
Stage 2 (Moderate)	160–179	100–109
Stage 3 (Severe)	180–209	110–119
Stage 4 (Very severe)	%210	%120

From the Joint National Committee on Detection, Evaluation, and Treatment of Hypertension, 1993

pressure affects 35 to 45 percent of women. Left untreated, high blood pressure can result in a stroke, heart attack, kidney damage, or vision problems.

A recent concept has emerged regarding hypertension in the elderly. Isolated systolic hypertension, which means high systolic readings with normal diastolic readings, are clinically significant.

Elderly women and men with systolic readings of 160 and normal diastolic measurements have a marked increase in the stroke and heart attack incidents.

Up to now, most of us took little heed in moderate isolated systolic hypertension, readings of 160 in the older person.

A recently completed major study, called the Systolic Hypertension in the Elderly Program (SHEP), proved the value of lowering isolated systolic hypertension in the elderly for the prevention of heart attacks and strokes. Yale was one of the major study centers.

DIAGNOSING HYPERTENSION. Despite the ease of accurately measuring someone's blood pressure, there are many gray areas in the diagnosis of hypertension. One casual blood pressure reading cannot diagnose hypertension. Measuring blood pressure on two or three different occasions can differentiate steady hypertension from labile hypertension, a condition in which blood pressure goes up and down throughout the day.

Some people's blood pressure is elevated only at work. A twenty-four-hour blood pressure monitoring device worn by the patient can detect this situation.

Blood pressure can be influenced by an individual's mood or level of stress. Some patients have high blood pressure only in the doctor's office, a syndrome known as white-coat hypertension. If the blood pressure is high on the first reading, the patient should sit quietly for a few minutes, or even lie down on the examining table, and have the reading repeated. The systolic blood pressure reading can vary from minute to minute. Seeing their blood pressure change so swiftly puzzles many patients. I explain to them that a simple increase in pulse rate can make the heart work harder and raise the blood pressure, and then it can quickly return to a healthy 120/70. Elevated blood pressure during times of stress is normal.

Generally, blood pressure is at its lowest level during the wee hours of the morning. Blood pressure begins to rise between 6 and 8 A.M. and can go higher or lower throughout the day. Pressure begins to fall toward midnight.

There is no ideal time to measure blood pressure. If any reading is abnormally high, it's wise to schedule several more readings at different times of the day. If a woman has normal blood pressure one day, and the next day her pressure rises to 139 systolic and 89 diastolic, a reading should be taken several additional times, at some regular interval. Fluctuating blood pressure may be a signal that her blood pressure is on the way to being permanently elevated.

CAUSES OF HYPERTENSION. Many patients wonder what has caused their hypertension. Unfortunately, we can find no direct cause in 90 percent of cases. The remaining 10 percent have a narrowing of the artery leading to the kidney (renal artery stenosis), a kidney disorder, or a rare tumor of the adrenal gland. Birth control pills sometimes spur hypertension, but it is reversible if the pill is discontinued. The pill is more likely to cause hypertension in women who are overweight and have a family history of high blood pressure.

For reasons that are as yet unclear, obesity can produce hypertension, as can too much alcohol. Drinking more than four ounces of alcohol a day is a significant cause of hypertension in both men and women.

We also know that hypertension runs in families. If one or both your parents have hypertension, then you have a higher-than-usual risk of developing it, too. By controlling hypertension and taking other precautions, you can significantly reduce your risks for heart disease and stroke.

SYMPTOMS OF HYPERTENSION. Hypertension is often called "the silent killer" because so many hypertensives have no symptoms. In some cases, hypertension is discovered during a doctor's visit or blood pressure screening. In others, the first inkling of hypertension is very dramatic: when they have a stroke or a heart attack.

Too many women are unaware that they have hypertension until a calamity occurs. One of them was Diane, a fifty-three-year-old jogger who was training for the New York Marathon. As I was driving on a country lane one day, I found her sprawled on the side of the road. She was conscious. Her blood pressure was 230 systolic and 138 diastolic. A slender nonsmoker, Diane was nonetheless at risk for high blood pressure; both her parents had died of strokes resulting from hypertension.

Her sudden steep rise in blood pressure apparently came on the heels of a ten-mile run. For months, she felt a little light-headed after her more strenuous runs, which she attributed to runner's high. At rest, her blood pressure was normal. Diane was experiencing very unstable (labile) high blood pressure. Her blood pressure is now controlled with medications and frequently monitored. She still jogs, but not more than five miles a day. Five miles is not an arbitrary figure. It was determined through an exercise stress test, which set Diane's safe parameters for exertion.

Diane was lucky that she was found by a physician who was able to render immediate aid. Other women with high blood pressure are told by their own bodies to get help. Of the various symptoms of high blood pressure, periodic headaches are the most common. My mother knew her blood pressure was on the rise when her head began pounding like a drum. Some mornings, she'd have a terrible ache in the back of her head, which made her reach for the valerian drops at her bedside. (Valerian drops were a mild sedative prescribed for hypertension because there was nothing else available in 1940.)

Among female hypertensives, headaches are sometimes accompanied by a feeling of uneasiness. This is especially true during menopause when the estrogen level begins to fall. Some menopausal women with high blood pressure say: "I feel as if my head is going to blow off."

While high blood pressure can cause headaches, nosebleeds are rare, contrary to popular belief. If the blood pressure rises to severe heights—over 250 systolic and 130 diastolic—blurred vision and severe headaches, not nosebleeds, will usually ensue. Extreme high blood pressure that comes on suddenly—malignant hypertension—requires emergency treatment because of the heightened risk of a heart attack or stroke.

HYPERTENSION AND PREGNANCY. Hypertensive women who become pregnant need expert care to prevent the serious complication of very high blood pressure, or eclampsia. Eclampsia is characterized by seizures and can lead to kidney failure and maternal or fetal death. A recent finding reported in *The New England Journal of Medicine* recommended that pregnant hypertensives take a daily dose of simple aspirin with no combinations to prevent eclampsia. Since there may be side effects produced by taking aspirin, such as stomach irritation or ulcers, hypertensive pregnant women should first consult their obstetricians before taking any drugs.

TREATING HYPERTENSION. Control hypertension and you are on the way to preserving good health. In the past twenty years, for example, the incidence of stroke has decreased by some 40 percent thanks largely to the aggressive treatment of hypertension.

Unfortunately, controlling hypertension is not easy. The goal is to keep blood pressure within the normal range most, if not all, of the time. The first step is knowing what your blood pressure is, just as you know your age and weight. Since a person's average blood pressure changes with each decade of life, it's important to have your pressure measured on a fairly regular basis. As we get older, our blood pressure rises. Our arteries become stiffer. They lose their flexibility and elasticity (arteriosclerosis), and the formerly glistening walls of the vessels are replaced by fibrous tissue. These changes alone result in some rise in the systolic blood pressure.

Another contributing factor is the body's increasing sensitivity to sodium (table salt). Before beginning any treatment for hypertension, your doctor should take a thorough dietary history. An important question that needs to be asked is: How much salt are you taking in each day?

Salt, which maintains life in all types of cells, is poison in excess quantities for many hypertensive people. It is not a universal dictum that all humans should avoid salt, but for many patients, salt causes hypertension to escalate.

Most people have a general notion of where the salt crystals are most abundant: salted crackers, soy sauce, anchovies, pretzels, salted popcorn, potato chips, pickles, pickled herring, and other delights. Seemingly innocent foods, however, also may be packed with salt: olives, canned tuna, relish, ketchup, frankfurters, bouillon cubes, carbonated beverages, hamburgers and other fast-food fare, tomato juice, sauerkraut, sardines, and canned lima beans, to name a few. The kosher woman who uses salt to pull the last drop of blood out of her meats sometimes forgets she is eating (and serving) too much salt.

The renowned physician Dr. Walter Klempner, who practiced medicine at Mount Sinai Hospital in New York City during the early 1940s, placed his hypertensive patients on a simple rice diet and was often able to control their condition. As mentioned earlier, there were no drugs in those days to treat hypertension except sedatives such as phenobarbital and valerian drops. My mother became one of Dr. Klempner's patients. She loved to eat and detested the rice diet, but Dr. Klempner convinced her that she had no choice but to follow his advice. In six months, her blood pressure was under control.

Many professionals thought Dr. Klempner was a charlatan, yet it was obvious that most of his rice diet patients did well. The rice diet worked because it was totally salt-free. Even so, many years passed before the medical profession finally accepted his dietary plan as scientifically proven, and now, fifty years later, the rice diet is still being used at such places as Duke University, where Dr. Klempner ultimately practiced for many years.

Today there are dozens and dozens of medications approved to treat hypertension and doctors too often forget the importance of eliminating as much salt as possible from the diet as a first step before resorting to drugs. More specifically, salt should be limited to 1,000 mg to 3,000 mg a day—about as much salt as there is in a bowl of New England clam chowder and seven pretzels.

Weight reduction (if you're overweight) and limiting alcohol intake to no more than one ounce a day are other early steps to take when mild hypertension is diagnosed. Eliminating salt, losing weight, and curbing alcohol may be sufficient to keep the blood pressure within the 140 systolic/85–90 diastolic range. These steps can reduce the blood pressure by 1 to 10 points systolic and 2 to 8 points diastolic. Even if you can keep your pressure down without medication, it's essential to have your blood pressure checked at least once a month.

In moderate to severe hypertension (160–170 systolic and 110–115 or higher diastolic), the patient is advised to further restrict salt intake, urged more strongly to lose weight, and is put on medication. These patients should be given an exercise stress test to determine how much exercise they can do safely. Only then can the doctor prescribe a sensible exercise program.

Scrupulously adhering to a low-salt, low-calorie diet and exercising at least three times a week for about twenty minutes per session can be a challenge, especially to a busy woman accustomed to a particular lifestyle. But these lifestyle changes are well worth the trouble because they may enable her to avoid medications, which are costly and may cause adverse side effects. If lifestyle changes alone fail to adequately lower the blood pressure after four weeks, medications usually become necessary.

TREATING HYPERTENSION WITH MEDICATION. To be sure, blood pressure medications have prevented countless heart attacks and strokes since they were developed in the 1950s. However, these drugs are ineffective and potentially dangerous if they are not taken as prescribed.

The most common reason blood pressure medication fails is simply because the patients don't take the prescribed dosage consistently. Research has shown that compliance for taking most prescription medications is poor, especially if more than one medication is needed. Some patients stop taking their medications because of the expense; others feel they cannot tolerate the side effects. And some simply forget to take it, especially if they have no symptoms of high blood pressure. Too many patients, once they run out of the medication, don't renew the prescription for weeks, or ever. These patients must be made to understand that it takes time for the medications to work. Hypertension is not controlled overnight.

Patients must also be aware that no drug can control hypertension effectively and still be free of potential adverse side effects. Fortunately, side effects occur in only 3 to 5 percent of users.

Sometimes, the patient will try different kinds of medication or set of medications before finding a regimen that is most effective and best tolerated. Everybody is different, so the medication taken by your sister may not be appropriate for you. The control of high blood pressure requires time. Medications cannot work overnight. Sometimes it takes many weeks, even months before the medication takes effect. You should not get discouraged if weeks go by and the blood pressure is not normal. Be patient!

Diuretics, also known as water pills, bring on frequent urination, which helps your body get rid of salt and excess water. Diuretics cause the blood vessels to dilate, lowering the blood pressure. Diuretics may be all you need to control your hypertension, if you couple it with weight loss, moderate exercise, and a low-salt, low-fat diet. Diuretics are especially useful for isolated hypertension.

Diuretics must be used with caution because they cause loss of potassium and magnesium, an increase in blood sugar in diabetics, and can bring on an attack of gout.

Beta-blockers are an excellent group of medications for the control of hypertension and angina (chest pain). These drugs block the formation of adrenaline-like substances. They particularly benefit those women who have rapid heartbeats and suffer from anxiety and hypertension. Beta-blockers can be given in conjunction with diuretics.

The downside of beta-blockers is they sometimes cause fatigue, but women are less vulnerable than men to this side effect. Beta-blockers also can decrease libido in some women. Women who suffer from depression should avoid beta-blockers because these drugs can deepen or prolong the depression. Overall, beta-blockers seem better tolerated by women than by men, though some studies have contradicted this observation.

Calcium channel blockers, another new group of hypertension medications, block calcium's entrance into the cell. The most annoying side effects are ankle swelling, dizzy spells, and constipation, which occur in some patients. If a women has varicose veins and swelling of the ankles, calcium channel blockers can make the swelling worse. If she suffers from chronic constipation, the drug verapamil, in particular, can aggravate the constipation.

Angiotensin-converting enzyme inhibitors, commonly known as ACE inhibitors, are also relatively recent and are very effective in lowering high blood pressure. But they certainly have their share of potential side effects, such as a chronic cough, dizzy spells, kidney failure, and, rarely, a precipitous drop in the blood pressure.

Among the other classes of medications used to combat hypertension are vasodilators, which dilate the blood vessels, and alpha-blocking agents, which in turn block the receptors that cause the blood vessels to narrow. These drugs' side effects may include dizzy spells, headaches, and weakness.

As a woman grows older and her arteries become stiffer, it often becomes increasingly difficult to control her high blood pressure. Two, three, and sometimes four different medications may be required. The more medications a person takes, the greater the possibility of side effects, and the less likely the patient is to take each pill at the right time. It is often necessary to change medications to find the right combination.

Sometimes the patient is overmedicated, and the blood pressure becomes too low. If this happens, the patient may experience dizzy spells because there is not enough pressure to get a sufficient blood supply to the brain. The woman might misinterpret dizziness as a sign that hypertension has returned, or she may even fear an impending stroke. Often, she will not share this symptom with her doctor. Failing to keep your doctor appraised of all your symptoms can be dangerous. Regardless of what medications are used, it is crucial that the patient and doctor work as a team to control hypertension.

One of the more common reasons I have been called to examine patients in the emergency room is because they nearly fainted or collapsed at home because their blood pressure fell too low. Many of these patients are elderly women who are taking highly effective blood pressure medications, which unfortunately tend to accumulate in the body and cause untoward reactions after prolonged use. A case in point is beta-blockers, which can cause the pulse rate to slow and make a person faint.

A doctor can sometimes predict the adverse effects of blood pressure drugs during each office visit by measuring the pulse rate and recording the blood pressure while the patient is sitting and standing. If the blood pressure falls when the person stands up, or if the pulse is becoming too slow, it is time to adjust the dosage. Several dosage adjustments may be necessary over a period of time.

Prescribing the right treatment has been further complicated by the commercialization of certain prescription drugs. These advertisements can confuse a patient and undermine her doctor's credibility, which adds to the difficulty of controlling hypertension.

Many times, patients have told me that their medication isn't working too well, and they ask me to prescribe a new drug they saw advertised on television. Often, these patients are surprised when I tell them they are already taking the advertised pill, but it is sold under a different name.

When the prescribed medication does not lower the blood pressure sufficiently, it could stem from the patient's failure to take the proper dosage, her failure to adequately curb her salt intake, or it may mean that she needs to add another medication.

On the flip side, some patients do so well on their medications that their doctor is able to wean them off the drugs entirely. I will frequently decrease the dosage slowly if the patient's pressure becomes normal and stays within normal limits, so long as she has her pressure checked at least once a month. Before reducing the dosage, I make sure the woman has lost weight if she was overweight, eliminated salt from her diet, started an exercise program, and taken steps to reduce her level of stress.

If the blood pressure is about 120 systolic and 80 diastolic during three consecutive visits to my office, I may decrease the medication to the smallest dosage possible. I reserve the right to increase the dosage if the pressure rises again in the future, but my aim is always governed by the same principle: fewer pills are better than more, and no pills are better than fewer pills—if the patient's natural internal pharmacy can keep the pressure in check.

For some patients, the disappearance of a stressful situation may extinguish the hypertension: the divorce is settled, business improves, the grieving for a loved one is over, there is a good job change, or the supervisor who made life miserable quits or gets fired.

One cardinal rule is: Don't stop taking the medication on your own, and do not wait until Saturday night to discover that you have taken your last pill, and then wait until Monday, or later, to refill the prescription. Withdrawing blood pressure medication abruptly can cause the pressure to suddenly rise to dangerous levels, resulting in a stroke.

FAMILY HISTORY

It is unclear how strong a role heredity plays in heart disease. You may fear you are at high risk if one or both of your parents died of a heart attack. It's entirely possible, however, that their attacks occurred because they were smokers and were overweight.

In a minority of families, many members die of coronary disease at a relatively young age. In most of these cases, the family members suffer from a congenital abnormality called familial hypercholesteremia, which causes the blood cholesterol level to soar. Today, much can be done with drugs and through surgery to save these individuals from premature death. In my practice I treat several families with familial hypercholesteremia. So far, some of these family members have reached the age of seventy and are still going strong.

ETHNIC AND SOCIOECONOMIC RISK FACTORS

There are inconclusive and confusing data on whether race plays a role in heart-disease risk. Many regions of China boast low heart-attack rates. But that is probably because their diet consists mainly of rice, vegetables, and complex carbohydrates. When Chinese adopt an American diet, their heart-attack rate equals ours.

Generally, people who immigrate to the United States from countries with low heart-attack rates may experience an increase in heart attacks if they adopt not only the typical hamburger/fried chicken–laden American diet, but some of our sedentary habits and workplace stresses as well.

African-Americans suffer from more hypertension and are more prone to heart attacks than the white population. Is it because blacks are generally poorer and therefore have less access to medical care? Is it because they tend to eat more salty foods and cook with less expensive saturated fats such as lard? Is it because of some genetic biological differences? We cannot make any sweeping generalizations about ethnicity and heart-disease risks until solid studies are completed.

In my practice, however, it is painfully evident that poor women of all races who live alone have a higher death rate from heart attacks than those who do not live alone. Surveys have shown that more than 50 percent of older people live alone. Since women generally outlive men, the majority of senior citizens living alone are women.

The elderly woman who lives alone and is poor almost never receives adequate medical care. She often lacks the ability—and the motivation—to get into an exercise program, especially during the winter months. Many older women lack mobility even in warm weather because they cannot drive. An older woman may reside in the inner city and therefore be afraid to take a brisk walk around her block. Most cook for themselves, and they may be unable to afford fresh vegetables, fish, and other healthful foods.

If they have meager pensions or live solely on Social Security, these women probably cannot afford to buy the expensive medications needed to keep their hearts and blood pressure under control. Some cardiac and blood pressure prescriptions cost up to $300 or $500 a month. Medicare generally does not cover prescriptions, although some states have programs to help qualifying seniors buy prescribed medications. If I and my colleagues didn't give out samples, I am sure that many of our patients would take no medications at all.

Many poor, elderly patients, both single and married, land in the emergency room because there were too many hurdles to overcome to take their medications consistently. Most are too proud to admit they cannot afford a doctor's visit or accept free care when we offer it to them.

Younger women also fall victim to heart disease (and other illnesses) because they cannot afford preventive medical care. This is especially true for uninsured divorced or single mothers who earn too much to qualify for Medicaid but not enough to buy health insurance.

HYPOTENSION

Some cardiologists once thought that blood pressure could never be too low. We now know that it can be. Statistically, hypotension—abnormally low blood pressure—generally spells longevity. Realistically, the condition can be dangerous because it can lead to fatigue, dizziness, and fainting.

In Victorian times, fainting was fashionable. It even gave rise to the swooning couch and smelling salts. It's no wonder, considering the tightly cinched waists that women wore in those days.

Swooning, fainting, and dizzy spells caused by hypotension can limit the kinds of jobs a person can safely hold. It also can prevent the patient from driving and restrict her life in a host of other ways. In some people, however, hypotension causes no problems at all. For example, young females in their teens, twenties, or thirties tend to run low blood pressures naturally. My daughters, ages thirty and thirty-two, both have blood pressure readings below 100 systolic and suffer no ill effects. If the drop in blood pressure is sudden enough to cause fainting, the condition is called orthostatic hypotension.

A reflex nervous response to an unpleasant situation or to pain, called a vago-vagal attack, is the most common cause of a temporary drop in blood pressure. Certain medications, including cardiac drugs and blood pressure pills, also can lead to hypotension. There are many other causes, such as heart attacks, bleeding, overwhelming infections, and genetics, that can make blood pressure too low. And there are medical causes, albeit rare, which need to be researched.

Another cause of debilitating low blood pressure can be a strict low-sodium diet.

Postprandial hypotension, the sudden loss of blood

pressure occurring after a meal, is particularly common among the elderly.

In most hypotension cases, though, no cause is found. The condition is usually cured simply by increasing the fluid and salt intake.

Other ways hypotensive patients can increase their blood pressure is by wearing elastic stockings or an old-fashioned girdle. If the woman continues to suffer frequent episodes of weakness or fainting, medications may be indicated.

PSYCHOLOGICAL FACTORS

Anger and frustration can precipitate a heart attack in both men and women. Rage, in particular, is a nonproductive emotion that forces the pulse to run wild, the blood pressure to rise suddenly, and places a strain on the heart. Rage arouses the adrenal glands to secrete more adrenaline, which, in turn, can trigger the arteries to go into spasms. This makes the blood more vulnerable to clotting. If a blood clot lodges in a coronary artery or the brain, a heart attack or stroke can ensue.

Many women have good reason to be angry. Most still earn less money per hour than their male counterparts, even if they work just as hard and are just as productive. Many divorced mothers get miserly alimony checks or fall victim to deadbeat dads. They become so deeply rooted in a lower economic soil, escape is almost impossible.

Two of my female patients suffered nasty divorces and, thanks to poor legal advice, received ridiculously low settlements while their husbands somehow managed to retain most of their estates. Both of these women suffered heart attacks after their divorce. The kind of anger these women experienced can cause the heart to speed into rapid, irregular rhythms and lead to cardiac arrest in someone whose coronary arteries were already narrowed.

After they recovered, I volunteered to appear in court on their behalf to ask for a more equitable settlement. In each case, a male judge refused to reconsider the settlements, ostensibly for legal reasons.

Another psychological risk factor is panic attacks, also known as anxiety attacks. Panic attacks, which usually occur early in the morning, produce major metabolic changes. Victims break into a sweat, their heart races out of control, their blood pressure rises; and if there is underlying heart disease, a heart attack may occur. In this sense, panic disorder is a scream for help.

Panic attacks can be triggered by a multitude of causes: an important test, giving a speech, financial distress, the threat of losing a home or friends, the fear of being alone or dying alone. Some panic attacks are based on unrealistic fears; others have no apparent trigger at all. Each of us has a demon or two that periodically surfaces and can manifest as panic. Whether these episodes qualify as panic disorder is a question of degree and frequency.

People who are disabled by their panic disorders need psychiatric counseling and medication. Panic disorder can usually be controlled or even cured by psychotherapy and drugs, such as tranquilizers and beta-blockers.

Treating chronic, debilitating anger is another matter. It often requires intense psychotherapy and a major change in attitude.

CHAPTER 4

HEART ATTACK: DIAGNOSIS AND TREATMENT

A heart attack can strike anywhere, day or night, at rest, at work, or at play. One minute the heart is receiving enough blood to function properly. The next minute, a blood clot, or thrombus, forms in one or more of the coronary arteries, blocking the flow of blood to the heart muscle. This is a heart attack.

Whether you survive the attack depends on many things: Did you recognize the early warning signs of a heart attack? Is someone nearby able to call an ambulance, or better yet, perform CPR (cardiopulmonary resuscitation) if your heart stops beating? How advanced was your heart disease before the heart attack? How close are you to an emergency room?

As explained in Chapter 2, it can be trickier for a woman to recognize heart-attack symptoms because many women—especially younger women—do not suffer the gripping chest pain so common among men. But some women do experience what's known as the "classical" heart-attack symptoms. Typically, these symptoms begin with a sudden crushing pain in the chest. The pain may radiate down the arm, up to the jaw, or to the upper back. The pain is usually accompanied by sweating and a feeling of impending doom. In many cases, the pain occurs during or after physical exertion, the arrival of bad news, or an unusually stressful event at work or at home.

Pain from a heart attack can awaken a person from a sound sleep. Says one heart-attack survivor: "It was as though a sledgehammer hit my chest." If you have been suffering from angina but now the pain persists, or it becomes greater in intensity, a heart attack may be in the making.

Most heart attacks happen between the early-morning hours and noon. Scientists speculate that this pattern may be tied to the body's internal clock and the types of hormones secreted at different times of the day. In the morning, the hormonal output is such that blood clots form easier and faster than at other times of the day. Also, people with panic disorders tend to suffer panic attacks in the early-morning hours. As noted in Chapter 3, a panic attack can trigger a heart attack in people with established heart disease.

Because men tend to experience the classic symptoms, they usually know when they are having a heart attack. Women, unfortunately, usually do not know. Aside from suffering unexpected heart-attack symptoms, many women have been brainwashed to think that a heart attack is a male affliction. They don't even consider the possibility of a heart attack when they have chest pain or the other types of pain described in Chapter 2.

Recognizing heart-attack symptoms can be difficult for doctors, too. According to the Quality Assurance Report, published by Physicians Health Services and issued to doctors in 1993, 25 percent of heart attacks are not recognized by doctors. This means that each year as many as forty thousand heart-attack victims are initially misdiagnosed, and most of them are women.

Of 7,700 male and female heart-attack patients in the Physicians Health Services study, 17 percent did not have typical chest pain, 35 percent had no pressure pains in the chest, 45 percent did not perspire, 25 percent complained of pain in the stomach, and 10 percent were relieved with antacids.

In the elderly patients, chest pain was reported in only 20 to 50 percent of the cases. Anxiety reactions and hyperventilation may mask heart attacks, especially in women, the study revealed.

Too often, people write off heart-attack pain as indigestion. Ignoring the symptoms, or denying that something life-threatening may be going on, is why about 85 to 90 percent of heart-attack deaths occur before the patient reaches the hospital. Of patients who get to the hospital alive, almost 85 percent survive.

Simply acknowledging that women are susceptible to heart attacks can be a lifesaver. Once a blood clot forms, every minute becomes precious. If the victim can be rushed to the hospital within six hours of the attack's onset, she is more likely to benefit from medications that dissolve the clot, and she is more likely to survive.

RAISING YOUR CHANCES OF SURVIVING A HEART ATTACK

Ideally, the heart-attack victim should be transported by ambulance with trained personnel at her side. If you live in a rural area or your address is not clearly marked on your mailbox, an ambulance might have difficulty finding your home. Ambulance drivers have been known to lose their way in the dark when there are few signposts to guide them. I instruct all my patients with heart disease to be able to relay the precise route to their home to the nearest fire company or ambulance squad. It can be helpful to write everything down and keep it near the phone as part of your "heart-attack survival kit." It's easy to forget the obvious during a life-or-death emergency.

After calling an ambulance, call your doctor and take simple aspirin. Aspirin makes the blood less sticky, preventing further clotting. If you are fortunate enough not to be alone at the time of the attack, ask the person with you to call 911 or your local emergency phone number.

Emergency medical technicians can transmit an ECG reading to the emergency room physician, who can order life-saving medicines to either speed up the heart rate or slow it down. Ambulance personnel are skilled in cardiopulmonary resuscitation (CPR), which can revive you if your heart has stopped and keep you alive en route to the hospital. Because the heart can stop at any time during a heart attack, it is more dangerous to take a patient to the hospital in a private car, but sometimes there is no choice.

Once you arrive in the emergency room, don't be afraid to ask the attending doctor: "Am I having a heart attack?" Be sure to say this loudly. This is especially important if you have high blood pressure, diabetes, a smoking habit, or you are overweight. If you are taken to a teaching hospital, the first doctor to examine you may be an intern with very little experience in diagnosing heart attacks. In any event, it can't hurt to remind doctors that men do not have a monopoly on heart attacks or heart disease. If a heart attack is confirmed, the time of its onset will help determine your treatment.

CLOT-BUSTERS. The primary heart-attack treatment, thrombolysis, can stop a heart attack in its tracks by dissolving the clot. Thrombolysis has reduced the heart-attack death rate by 20 percent.

Although the most effective clot-busting drugs, streptokinase and TPA, did not come into their own until the late 1980s, thrombolysis is not a new idea. Fifty years ago, some doctors conceived the notion of dissolving blood clots using leeches. Leeches secrete a powerful clot-dissolving chemical called hirudin. Researchers at Yale School of Medicine and other medical centers are studying ways to use hirudin to develop new clot-dissolving drugs.

As with diagnostic tests, women are less likely than men to receive thrombolysis, according to one recent study called the Myocardial Infarction Triage and Intervention Trial (MITI). The reason, MITI found, was that women were less likely to meet the criteria for thrombolytic treatment than men. The most important criteria are: The heart attack must be less than six hours old, and there must be no recent history of internal bleeding since the treatment can cause life-threatening hemorrhages in the brain and gastrointestinal tract. Thrombolysis candidates also must have an abnormal ECG and best be under age seventy-five.

Emily, a computer specialist who smoked thin cigars that someone had told her were safer than cigarettes, could not benefit from thrombolysis because she didn't make it to the hospital until fourteen hours after her symptoms began.

Interviewed in the coronary care unit, Emily told the medical team what happened: "I've had indigestion at night for years, and my doctor warned me that my smoking and drinking would do me in. He prescribed an antacid, which I took nearly every evening. Then one night, after a pretty wild few hours of sex, alcohol, and cigars, I got a terrible case of heartburn and chest pain. I could not catch my breath. The pain would not go away with the antacid. I walked up and down my house all night, smoking more and becoming more short of breath. I really got scared when I felt my heart beating differently, racing as it never had before. My boyfriend rushed me to the ER of the local hospital. I can't even recall the rest, except that I woke up in the recovery room."

At age thirty-nine, Emily had suffered a severe heart attack. Her ECG showed a massive attack in the front of her heart (the anterior wall) as well as the back of her heart (the inferior wall). All three of her coronary arteries were blocked. Her heart was heavily damaged, but her condition improved after a coronary bypass operation.

Today, however, Emily is totally disabled. Someday soon, she may need a heart transplant. Her heart might have avoided severe damage and her quality of life would probably be vastly improved had she arrived at the hospital in time to receive thrombolysis.

Waiting too long to get to the hospital, as Emily did, is one of the primary reasons women are less likely to receive thrombolysis. Women delay seeking help because their heart-attack symptoms may not include chest pains. Their symptoms may instead include light-headedness, irregular heartbeats, shortness of breath, or pains in the jaw, shoulders, or arms. Forty percent of women over age seventy-five had no chest pain with their heart attacks.

Another reason fewer women get thrombolysis is doctors' fear that women with hypertension and diabetes are more susceptible to internal bleeding.

The age criteria also works against women. As many as 25 percent of heart-attack victims don't qualify for thrombolysis because of their advanced age, and women make up a significant portion of older heart-attack victims. Eighty-five percent of heart-attack deaths occur in people over age sixty-five. Fifty percent occur in those over age seventy-five, most of whom are women.

The age requirement was set because older patients tend to have poorer outcomes. The age criteria is controversial, however, and may be subject to change in the future. In Europe, patients over age eighty may qualify for thrombolytic treatment. In the United States, many cardiologists still believe the risk is too high for cerebral hemorrhage in patients over age seventy-five. In addition to reassessing the age criteria, researchers are looking into whether thrombolysis might still be useful after six hours of the heart attack's onset.

Without thrombolytic treatment, the heart-attack death rate is five times higher.

CHAPTER 5

DIAGNOSTIC TESTS FOR FEMALE HEART DISEASE

There are many different tests physicians use to diagnose heart disease. Some tests invade the body; others are noninvasive. Some are widely available; others are found only in a few medical centers around the country. Some tests are passive; others require you work hard enough to break a sweat. And some diagnostic tools work better with men than women. Which tests your doctor orders and how many will depend on your individual circumstances. This chapter will discuss each of the diagnostic tests currently being used to detect cardiac problems, beginning with the most basic tool: the stethoscope.

THE STETHOSCOPE

The stethoscope was invented by a young doctor named René Laennec in nineteenth-century France because he was tired of catching fleas from his patients. Before the stethoscope, doctors listened to the heart by placing an ear directly on a patient's bare chest. Aside from catching fleas, Laennec found this method to be rather embarrassing whenever he examined a young woman in the famous Nestlé hospital where he worked.

One day, Laennec rolled a magazine into a cylinder, placed it on the chest of a young woman, and heard her heart sounds clearly. He was ridiculed for using a cylinder to examine the heart. Oliver Wendell Holmes even wrote a mocking poem, called "The Stethoscope Song."

The modern stethoscope is more sophisticated, but uses the same principle to amplify heart sounds. It's the first and most important instrument the doctor uses to listen to the heart. A stethoscope can detect murmurs and other abnormal heart sounds as well as irregular heart rhythms. With the stethoscope, a doctor can even diagnose diseased valves. The stethoscope cannot, however, diagnose a heart attack or angina.

THE ELECTROCARDIOGRAM

Each time the heart beats, it is responding to an electrical stimulus generated within the cells of the heart muscle. The electrocardiogram, or ECG, is a machine capable of recording those electrical events. The ECG was developed by Dr. Willem Einthoven in the nineteenth century and was introduced in the United States by Paul Dudley White of Boston in the early part of this century.

At that time, the ECG machine was so big that it took up most of White's laboratory. Long cables led from the laboratory, down a flight of stairs, through the halls, to the patient's bedside. Today, the ECG weighs just a few pounds and can be hand-carried.

An ECG can diagnose a heart attack, a thickening of the heart (left ventricular hypertonic), and irregular heartbeats. An ECG tracing also can diagnose angina if the tracing is taken during the pain.

An ECG reading can be misleading. In the early hours of a heart attack, for example, the ECG is normal in about 25 percent of cases. Some women have silent ischemia (too little blood and oxygen going to the heart) without any symptoms. A portable ECG, called a Holter monitor, worn by the patient over a twenty-four-hour period can sometimes detect silent ischemia, also known as silent angina. Silent ischemia can lead to a heart attack and sudden death.

EXERCISE STRESS TEST

To diagnose the origin of chest pain arising from the heart, and to confirm the presence of angina or silent ischemia, doctors depend on the exercise stress test.

During strenuous exercise, the heart has to work five times harder than it does at rest, and it must be able to pump adequate oxygen-rich blood to the heart muscle. To make oxygen delivery possible, the coronary arteries must be open. If, during exercise, insufficient oxygen arrives at the heart muscle, it becomes pale and ischemic. An ECG taken at that moment will register an abnormal pattern, called an ischemic pattern. At that point, the patient may experience chest pain.

Dr. Arthur Master of New York devised the first exercise stress test in the late 1940s. Leads were attached from a patient to an electrocardiogram, which recorded the electrical impulses while the patient stepped up and down on a two-step ladder. The ladder has since been replaced by a stationary bicycle or treadmill.

The first step is to determine a target heart rate, which is calculated according to the patient's age. The younger the patient, the faster the heart must beat to achieve diagnostic value. If the patient is able to exercise only enough to elevate her pulse to 100, the ECG might be unable to tell whether her coronary arteries are blocked or narrowed, unless she happens to display changes in her ECG tracing at that level.

People who have never used a treadmill or are otherwise unaccustomed to exercise often cannot perform the exercise stress test. Nor can patients who suffer from lung disease, because their lung capacity is inadequate. Although some sedentary women can use a stationary bike with ease, the bicycle can be difficult for older or obese women, and those with back problems.

In many cases, older women aren't given the option of taking an exercise stress test because their ECG is normal and their pain is not focused in their chest. As mentioned in Chapter 1, this is a common reason why coronary artery blockages in older women are often not diagnosed in a timely manner.

WHO SHOULD HAVE A STRESS TEST? There are many reasons for women to have a stress test. But the HMOs, Medicare, Medicaid, and other insurance companies do not always pay for it, and doctors may not order it for that reason alone. Some insurers that preach prevention will refuse to pay for a routine exercise stress test, even for high-risk patients. These patients include postmenopausal women with high triglycerides, low HDL, and high LDL; smokers; diabetic women; women with high blood pressure; and those with a strong family history of heart attacks.

All these women may have coronary artery disease that is silent, and unless it is identified, these women may become another statistic. The irony is that diagnoses made possible through stress testing can help lower women's heart-attack risk and very often prevent heart attacks and sudden death—ultimately saving the insurance companies and Medicare billions of dollars.

Another reason for having a stress test is to confirm a diagnosis of angina and to determine its seriousness. Women who suffer from unusual chest pains must have a cardiac stress test, and anyone who has an abnormal resting ECG also should have a stress test, along with other cardiac testing, to determine the cause.

It is customary to order an exercise stress test after a heart attack while the patient is still in the hospital, and periodically after bypass operations or balloon dilatations of blocked arteries (balloon angioplasty).

Exercise stress tests also can be performed to determine a heart patient's capacity for exercise. Some cardiologists use stress tests to gauge the effectiveness of medications the patient is taking to treat hypertension or irregular heart actions.

If, during the exercise stress test, the patient experiences shortness of breath, chest pain, irregular heart rhythms, or other severe ECG changes, the test is discontinued.

Blood pressure must be meticulously monitored during the test. If it falls, this is yet another danger signal to stop the test. It could mean that there is dangerous blockage of the coronary arteries or it could be a reflexive drop in pressure (a vago-vagal attack). A drop in pressure during the test also can stem from dehydration or from medications the patient is taking. Even fear of the test itself can cause the blood pressure to fall.

It is rare that the test can trigger a heart attack, and rarer still that it can precipitate sudden death. In one survey of exercise stress tests, a mortality rate of 1 per 100,000 was reported.

A stress test should not begin while the patient is having chest pain because it could mean their angina has progressed to a heart attack. Under this circumstance, a stress test could be disastrous.

The test is considered positive (meaning abnormal) if there are ECG changes, described as ST waves, drifting above or below the baseline of the recording, regardless of whether chest pain is present. A positive test usually means the coronary arteries are more than 75 percent blocked. Arteries with a 50 percent blockage are potentially troublesome, but they usually are not revealed by the stress test.

Exercise stress test results can be negative if only one blood vessel is diseased, and single-vessel disease is more common in women than in men. If all three coronary arteries are blocked by more than 75 percent, the majority of women will show a positive result.

A positive stress test can be very difficult to interpret in women. ST-segment changes that dip below the baseline do not necessarily indicate that the arteries are blocked. These are called false-positive changes and are most common in young women. In many such cases, we cannot deduce that a positive stress test in women identifies blocked arteries, and we must look further.

Mitral valve prolapse syndrome (see Chapter 6) also can produce false-positive changes, as can rapid breathing and a low potassium level in the blood. A potassium deficiency can result from diuretics that many women take for bloating, swelling of the ankles, or to lose weight. Unfortunately, some pharmacists automatically renew diuretic prescriptions without checking with the doctor. Bulimia (forced gorging and purging) and abuse of enemas also may be responsible for low potassium, which may not only cause false-positive stress tests, but can lead to dangerous heart rhythms and sudden death.

Digitalis (foxglove), which improves cardiac function, also can produce false-positive stress tests. Properties of the foxglove plant bear a very strong similarity to estrogen. Researchers speculate that the high percentage of false-positive stress tests in older women may stem from estrogen-replacement therapy since estrogen resembles digitalis—a theory that will require much more data before it can be accepted by the medical community.

Despite the fact that the exercise stress test has less diagnostic value in women than in men, it is still a good tool for diagnosing coronary artery disease. The test should always be administered by an experienced doctor and not solely by technicians.

THALLIUM STRESS TEST

A more complicated and costly version of the exercise stress test employs thallium, a radioactive isotope. A positive thallium stress test suggests that one or more arteries of the heart are blocked. Cardiac catheterization (described later in this chapter) should be considered if there are widespread abnormalities on the thallium exercise stress test.

Joyce, a thirty-eight-year-old schoolteacher who suffered from recurrent chest pain, was given a thallium stress test after a regular stress test turned up positive.

Even though Joyce was a nonsmoker, her physician ordered the thallium test because both her parents had died of heart disease. A regular stress test is given first in hopes that a definitive diagnosis can be reached. Only when there is a potentially false-positive result will the thallium version be ordered.

"Why bother with a simple stress test if it has so many false-positive results?" Joyce asked her physician.

A thallium stress test requires two gamma cameras (nuclear scan cameras), her doctor explained. The radioactive thallium is specially ordered for each test and must be used within twenty-four hours. A specialist in nuclear medicine, a cardiologist, nuclear medicine technicians, and in some settings, a physicist, all are involved. The nuclear waste material requires special handling. All this elevates the cost of a thallium stress test to $500 to $1,500—two to three times more than a simple stress test.

The thallium test takes up most of the day, but it has about a 90 percent chance of being accurate if the arteries are more than 75 percent blocked. If a patient is unable to exercise, a rest exercise is performed, which is called a persantine thallium stress test.

In some ways, Joyce found that the thallium test was identical to the simple exercise stress test. At the peak of her exercise, though, the doctor injected thallium into an IV that had been put in her arm before the test began. If her arteries were clear, the thallium would be evenly distributed through her heart. Her doctor, highly skilled in the procedure, knew that a woman's breasts can sometimes obscure the appearance of thallium distribution, so he read the gamma scans accordingly.

Fortunately, the thallium test was normal, in spite of the previously abnormal stress test. As a backup measure, Joyce also had an echocardiogram (described in the next section), which was normal, too.

Soon after taking the tests, Joyce's chest pains disappeared. Their cause remains a mystery.

THE ECHOCARDIOGRAM

Echocardiography (also known as sonography or ultrasound) is used in medical centers throughout the country to evaluate the heart during a stress test. Instead of scanning the heart that has been bathed in a radioactive isotope, the echocardiogram uses sound waves to create a visual image. Relatively inexpensive, echocardiography is the safest and least psychologically threatening heart exam a patient can undergo. Free of side effects and aftereffects, echocardiography can be repeated hundreds of times in the same patient.

When I started in the cardiology field twenty-five years ago, one of my colleagues, now a prominent cardiologist, called echocardiograms a Rorschach test, the ink blots used in psychological testing. At that time, the cardiac images made no sense at all to the uninitiated and were difficult to evaluate even with experience. As the technique became more refined, we began getting an image of the heart and valves as faithful as those that might appear if we were to open the chest and peek inside.

We learned the principle of ultrasound from dolphins and bats, who emit sound waves that bounce back and give the animal its bearings. During World War I, electronic sound waves sent to the depths of the ocean detected German submarines. The ultrasound technique has since been adapted to evaluate the heart and other internal organs.

Echocardiography is now used as routinely as the ECG, but it requires expensive equipment and an expertly trained, experienced physician to perform the examination properly.

With modern echocardiography, doctors can observe the heart muscle contract and relax before, during, and after the patient walks on a treadmill or rides a stationary bicycle. The heart's chambers and valves also can be visualized. Unlike the thallium test, however, the echocardiogram cannot clearly show the coronary arteries. But doctors know that if the heart is receiving a normal supply of blood, it contracts uniformly throughout the stress test. If the heart muscle is inadequately nourished, the contractions will be abnormal.

Echocardiography has technical limitations. If a patient has emphysema or is obese, for example, a noninvasive echocardiogram may not be possible. In order to overcome these limitations, we now can pass an echocardiographic probe (known as a transducer) through the mouth and into the esophagus to obtain a marvelously clear view of the contracting heart and its valves. Using a color monitor to pick up the bouncing sound waves, we can actually follow the flow of blood as it makes its way through the various crevices of the heart.

EQUILIBRIUM RADIONUCLIDE ANGIOCARDIOGRAM

The equilibrium radionuclide angiocardiogram (also known as the multigated graft acquisition or MUGA) is a nuclear imaging test, as is the thallium stress test. A short-lived radioactive isotope is injected into the patient. The gamma rays accumulated in the heart are scanned with a gamma camera and analyzed by a computer. The computer provides a numerical measurement of how well the heart is contracting and ejecting oxygenated blood to the rest of the body. The measurement is called the ejection fraction. A weakened heart muscle will yield a low ejection fraction.

A low ejection fraction may stem from blocked coronary arteries, muscle disease, congenital valve disease, tumors, or metabolic diseases, such as an underactive thyroid gland. The ejection fraction also can determine how severely injured a heart muscle is and help the doctor determine which medications to prescribe.

POSITRON EMISSION TOMOGRAPHY (PET)

Positron emission tomography is a relatively new research instrument that measures the metabolism of the heart. It basically is a more sophisticated and more expensive version of the MUGA. It currently is used on a research basis only but is being evaluated for routine use on cardiac patients.

PET tells the cardiologist how efficiently the heart utilizes its metabolic fuel—oxygen. PET also identifies areas of the heart that are not destroyed after a heart attack.

MAGNETIC RESONANCE IMAGING (MRI)

Magnetic resonance imaging is a remarkable diagnostic tool that uses magnets rather than X rays or sound waves to create a three-dimensional image of internal organs. Initially used to visualize the brain, MRI is now used to scan most any organ. When MRI is used to scan the heart, hundreds of crisp, detailed images can show any cardiac damage that might be present.

Recently at Beth Israel Hospital in Boston, Dr. Warren Manning used MRI to visualize the coronary arteries, a technique he dubbed "magnetic resonance angiography." Although magnetic resonance angiography is in its infancy, it may someday preclude the need for diagnostic cardiac catheterization, an invasive procedure used to visualize the coronary arteries (see next section).

At present, magnetic resonance angiography has some limitations. The patient must lie perfectly still for varying periods of time in an enclosed tunnel and endure the noisy moving of the magnets. Some patients become claustrophobic and cannot complete the test. Patients with pacemakers, artificial hips, or any metals on or in the body cannot undergo this test or the metal object will be moved out of position.

CARDIAC CATHETERIZATION AND ANGIOGRAPHY

The first cardiac catheterization was performed by a German surgeon, Dr. Werner Forssmann, in 1929 when he snaked a urinary catheter into his own heart. He won a Nobel prize for his feat in 1956 despite his earlier flirtations with the Nazi regime. In 1958, a group of physicians became the first to visualize the coronary arteries after they injected dye into a catheterized heart and took X rays. The technique was called angiography.

Today, cardiac catheterization coupled with angiography is considered the gold standard for diagnosing diseased coronary arteries. Its use has been widespread since 1980.

To understand cardiac catheterization, it helps to first know about the coronary arteries. There are two major vessels—a left artery and a right artery—that arise from the aorta, the heart's main artery. In general terms, the left artery supplies the front of the heart and the right artery feeds the back of the heart. The left artery quickly divides into the left anterior descending artery and the circumflex artery. The left anterior descending artery supplies the left side of the heart, and the circumflex artery supplies the wall that separates the right and the left sides of the heart. Severe blockage of any of these arteries jeopardizes the portions of the heart muscle they supply.

During cardiac catheterization, a long flexible tube called a catheter is passed by way of the artery in the arm or groin into a coronary artery. Once the catheter reaches the heart, dye is injected through the tube into the coronary arteries. Specialized X rays called angiograms are then taken. Partially sedated during the procedure, the patient feels a burning sensation when the dye is injected and may feel the tugging and pulling of the catheter.

The image resulting from the catheterization is so clear that the cardiologist can tell whether the coronary arteries are blocked and to what degree. The angiogram also serves as a road map that helps the doctor prescribe the best treatment to remedy the problem.

Cardiac catheterization is performed at least 500,000 times a year in the United States, mostly on men. In one study at St. Louis University, only 38 percent of women with abnormal exercise stress tests were given cardiac catheterization compared with a majority of the men. This disparity occurred despite the fact that the women had a fivefold increased risk of heart attack or death within the next two years. The St. Louis study further found that men underwent twice as many cardiac catheterization and coronary bypass surgeries as women who complained of angina or had abnormal thallium exercise stress tests.

I believe one of the primary reasons fewer women get cardiac catheterization is because their doctors simply do not refer them for the procedure as readily as they refer their male patients. Too many doctors continue to attribute a woman's cardiac symptoms to a psychosomatic illness.

In the following case, however, a cardiac catheterization proved that a patient's chest pains were not of cardiac origin.

Josephine became my patient when she switched HMOs. She already had been diagnosed with angina and was taking at least three medications to control her chest pains.

Josephine called me incessantly, claiming her chest pain was always a little different. In each case, the pain came on the heels of an argument with her husband, daughter, or somebody else.

"It feels like someone is pulling at my breast," she'd say one time. "It feels like someone stabbed me," she'd say the next. She was always asking for new medications because her old ones weren't helping anymore.

She refused to have an exercise stress test, and, at her own insistence, landed in the emergency room at least once a month. We finally convinced her to have a cardiac catheterization. To her surprise, she was found to have clear arteries, no spasms of the coronary arteries, and she did not have Syndrome X. There was no medical reason for her recurrent chest pain. For ten years, Josephine had been treated for an illness she did not have.

I was thrilled to be able to tell her that her arteries were normal, she had no angina, and her risk for a heart attack was no higher than the next healthy person's risk.

"Of course I have angina," she insisted. "Just ask my family how sick I am. I am switching doctors immediately. You are off my case."

The reason for her anger at me was obvious. Josephine used complaints of chest pains to win arguments with her family members, and here I was taking away the "illness" that she had relied on all those years.

To her credit, Josephine at least permitted us to perform a cardiac catheterization on her. Some women (as well as men) are too afraid; others fail to ask their doctors about cardiac catheterization because they do not know it is available.

Who, then, should get cardiac catheterization with angiography? There is universal agreement that it should be performed on patients with severe, well-documented angina; before, during, and after a heart attack if medications did not help; and in cases where balloon angioplasty or bypass surgery is planned.

Other reasons include a strong suspicion, based on tests described earlier in this chapter, that:

- A heart valve is narrowed or leaking, causing symptoms, and surgical repair is contemplated;
- Angina flares after a heart attack;
- Angina that is controlled with medication worsens;
- An exercise thallium stress test is clearly positive, and the woman suffers from chest pain; or
- The woman has chest pain, the exercise stress test is negative, but she has risk factors such as smoking, diabetes, high cholesterol, family history of heart disease, and she is postmenopausal.

Sometimes, cardiac catheterization is performed needlessly because doctors fear a lawsuit. Recently we saw a young, active woman who had chest pain and an abnormal thallium stress test without any risk factors. None of the cardiologists believed this woman had coronary artery disease. But we gave her a cardiac catheterization anyway. Not surprisingly, her arteries were normal, and she had no spasms of her coronary arteries (which sometimes cause chest pain). Our diagnosis of Syndrome X (see Chapter 2), which we reached before the catheterization, remained the same after the catheterization.

In a recent study from Boston, researchers estimated that 50 percent of coronary angiography procedures being done in the United States are "unnecessary, or at least could be postponed." These findings came from patients who sought second opinions before deciding whether to submit to catheterization. This study will need to be confirmed, however, before it can be convincing, because most cardiologists disagree with its findings.

CARDIAC CATHETERIZATION RISKS. Cardiac catheterization is a relatively safe procedure, but it is not free from potential complications. In rare instances, the procedure can cause strokes, hemorrhages, heart attacks, kidney failure, or death. Women who are obese, diabetic, or over age seventy are at greatest risk for complications, but these are the patients who are more likely to need catheterization because their heart-attack risk is elevated. Women with chronic kidney disease must understand that the dye used for angiography sometimes can cause the kidneys to shut down completely, and they may need renal dialysis for several months. With some of the newer dyes, this complication is less likely.

If you have any doubts before agreeing to a catheterization, seek a second opinion unless your life is in immediate danger. In a nonemergency situation, the second opinion should come from a "noninvasive cardiologist"—a cardiologist who does not perform catheterization.

The decision to do a cardiac catheterization should not be made quickly by you or your doctor. Be sure all your questions about the procedure and its risks are answered before you sign the consent form. Even if your cardiologist is well known in your community as an expert, he or she should still take the time to explain everything to you in terminology you understand.

Don't be overly frightened about the potential complications, though. It helps to remember that thousands of lives are saved each year thanks to cardiac angiography.

ULTRAFAST SCANNING

A new, noninvasive method is now being tested to visualize the coronary arteries without having to resort to cardiac catheterization. This painless procedure uses an Ultrafast scanner, which is actually a CAT scan of the coronary arteries. Ultrafast scanning can identify calcium deposits in the artery, which is a marker for coronary artery disease (atherosclerosis). The absence of calcium negates the need for cardiac catheterization because it virtually excludes the diagnosis of severe coronary artery disease in older women. Younger people can have some blockage of their arteries even without calcium deposits, however.

Ultrafast scanning is expected to become an excellent diagnostic tool for women who have abnormal results from standard and thallium exercise stress tests. It also may be an ideal screening tool for women at high risk for heart attack if subjected to cardiac catheterization.

I anticipate that Ultrafast scanners will be available in most hospitals before the end of this decade. The cost of this test should be a fraction of the cost of cardiac catheterization.

A CASE STUDY IN DIAGNOSING HEART DISEASE

Molly was a delightful seventy-nine-year-old grandmother when she became my patient. Twenty pounds overweight, Molly also has diabetes. Despite severe arthritis in her back and legs, she cooked, cleaned, and baby-sat each weekend for her ten grandchildren.

After her first great-granddaughter was born, Molly took charge, hobbling along in her usual loving way. But now she felt a terrible heaviness between her breasts each time she played actively with the infant. Molly knew what that feeling was all about. She remembered her husband complaining of the same feeling, but he was stubborn and refused to see a doctor. He passed away without ever seeking medical care.

Molly made an appointment with me immediately.

After listening to her heart through a stethoscope and hearing nothing abnormal, I ordered an ECG, which was abnormal.

A standard exercise stress test was impractical because Molly could neither walk on a treadmill nor ride a bicycle. Fortunately, patients like Molly can still have a stress test while lying on a table. This Persantine thallium stress test is as precise as a thallium stress test and is ideal for the patient with orthopedic problems or who is too frail to undergo the regular stress test.

Molly's Persantine test results indicated possible blockages in her coronary arteries. To gain more specific information, I ordered a cardiac catheterization, which showed that all three of her coronary arteries were blocked.

After a successful bypass operation, Molly is back to her favorite endeavor—baby-sitting, but now it's with her third great-grandchild.

CHAPTER 6

MITRAL VALVE PROLAPSE SYNDROME: "THE WOMAN'S DISEASE"

A line of patients is waiting in a medical station located in a tent somewhere in Verdun, France. The year is 1916. The American doctor, Samuel Levine, from Boston, is listening to their complaints.

"My heart is pounding like it's going to jump out of my chest," a tall, thin American soldier tells the doctor. "It hurts. I can't breathe. I feel weak, shaky, giddy, exhausted. I just can't go on."

The young infantryman has a frightened look on his face. His hands are cold, and he is perspiring. His physical examination is normal, and his heart sounds fine. But the doctor has heard the same complaints from dozens and dozens of others.

Dr. Levine dubs the condition "a soldier's heart." During the Civil War, another doctor had labeled it "neurocirculatory asthenia."

In 1994, female patients with the same set of symptoms often receive a diagnosis of "mitral valve prolapse syndrome." In some cases, the diagnosis is valid. In many other cases, it is not.

The mitral valve, shaped like a bishop's miter, separates the upper chamber of the heart—the left atrium—from the lower, more powerful chamber—the left ventricle. The valve acts like a traffic cop, opening to allow blood to flow from the upper to the lower chamber. Each time the valve snaps shut, it prevents blood from backing up in the wrong direction.

The valve is attached by leaflets and cords of tissue to the muscles of the left side of the heart. The valve looks like it is suspended by strings, like a marionette. If one or all of the leaflets bulges, or prolapses, into the upper chamber, the valve does not close completely, allowing blood to leak back into the atrium. As the valve bulges, it makes a clicking sound, and any leakage produces a murmur. That is why prolapse of the mitral valve is also called the click-murmur syndrome, the floppy-valve syndrome, or the balloon mitral valve.

The actual pathology of this condition was first demonstrated, through angiograms and autopsies, in 1963. People with congenital heart disease, rheumatic heart disease, coronary artery disease, or disease of the heart muscle may develop mitral valve prolapse. The precise cause is unknown.

In the past two decades since the introduction of echocardiography, several studies have suggested that 5 to 10 percent of all women suffer from mitral valve prolapse to some degree. These statistics may be inaccurate, however, because they were generated before echocardiography began using uniform criteria for diagnosis.

POSSIBLE COMPLICATIONS. The majority of people with mitral valve prolapse syndrome live a long, symptom-free life. But some patients do suffer complications.

The bulging leaflets connecting the valve to the heart muscle become a favorite place for bacteria to settle and proliferate. This condition, called endocarditis, can damage or destroy the valve and possibly kill the patient. Endocarditis is usually heralded by night sweats and fever caused by the valve becoming inflamed. Endocarditis can be prevented or treated with antibiotics.

A small percentage of women, especially as they become older, can rupture one of the prolapsed leaflets, which can result in a medical emergency. They may need a new valve.

Stroke is another potential complication of mitral valve prolapse. As the valve collects calcium on its surface, a small piece can dislodge, travel to the brain, and cause a small stroke, called a transient ischemic attack, or TIA.

Older medical textbooks describe the stereotypical woman suffering from mitral valve prolapse as being thin, flat-chested, anxious, hypertensive, and with above-average intelligence. Today, doctors realize that these characteristics were arbitrary, and there is no typical type of woman who has this disorder.

Sometimes, women experience symptoms that are consistent with mitral valve prolapse, but there is no proof that the condition is present. Some doctors will give the diagnosis anyway, just to appease the patient who is not satisfied if she is told nothing is wrong with her heart. Some patients will run to ten doctors until they get a diagnosis. These patients, both male and female, evidently prefer being told they are suffering from a heart abnormality than having to admit that their symptoms are psychosomatic.

More commonly, an echocardiogram reveals a slight prolapse of the mitral valve that needs no medical treatment. Nonetheless, a beta-blocker is frequently prescribed prematurely to ward off a fast heartbeat. The patient then gets stuck with the diagnosis of mitral valve prolapse and continues taking a drug that she does not need.

SYMPTOMS OF MITRAL VALVE PROLAPSE

Many times, floppy valve syndrome produces no symptoms. The disorder may be found by chance during a routine physical examination.

When symptoms are present, they sometimes take the form of palpitations, rapid or irregular heart rhythms, and chest pain. Panic reactions, dizziness, feeling faint, and shortness of breath all may be associated with mitral valve prolapse. If a patient with these symptoms had been treated with tranquilizers and undergone psychotherapy in the past, the doctor may think the symptoms are psychosomatic and miss the true diagnosis of mitral valve prolapse.

Chest pain caused by a floppy valve can appear while resting or during physical exertion. The type of chest pain can vary; it has been described as "sticking," "crushing," "pulling," "stabbing," and "nagging." The pain sometimes has the same characteristics as angina. An important aphorism I teach medical students is that an elephant can have both fleas and lice. Even if mitral valve prolapse is present, the chest pain could still be coming from diseased coronary arteries and not from the mitral valve. Both conditions can occur simultaneously, each giving rise to different symptoms.

If you have a firm diagnosis of mitral valve prolapse, call your doctor immediately should any of the following symptoms arise:

- Sudden shortness of breath;
- New chest pain;
- Dizzy spells or fainting episodes;
- Vision problems;
- Numbness or weakness; or
- Night sweats and fevers.

DIAGNOSING MITRAL VALVE PROLAPSE

I became interested in floppy valve syndrome about twenty years ago when echocardiography was in its infancy. I and my colleagues examined hundreds of women of all ages and found many with a slight prolapse of the mitral valve but no murmurs or clicks. Despite the slight prolapse, these women did not fulfill the criteria for the diagnosis.

If the prolapse is severe enough, the condition can be detected, or at least suspected, by listening to the heart through a stethoscope. The doctor will hear the characteristic click followed by a murmur. If the prolapse is slight, there may be no audible evidence.

If the doctor hears the click and murmur or has other reasons to suspect floppy valve syndrome, an echocardiogram should be ordered. Unless there is click and murmur and solid echocardiographic evidence of a ballooning mitral valve, the diagnosis should be abandoned.

If palpitations are one of the main symptoms, the patient should wear a Holter monitor—the portable, continuous electrocardiogram machine described in Chapter 5—for twenty-four or forty-eight hours. There are many types of normal and abnormal heart rhythms that can be detected by the Holter monitor. Sometimes, the monitor picks up no palpitations because they did not occur. The patient wearing the monitor can actually transmit her heartbeat through a telephone line to a central station for analysis whenever she feels her heart racing. If an abnormality is present, the best-suited medication can be prescribed to prevent those frightening sensations of a runaway heart rhythm.

A CASE OF MISTAKEN DIAGNOSIS. Unfortunately, the diagnosis of mitral valve prolapse is often made without good scientific evidence. Floppy valve syndrome is a convenient diagnosis to pin on patients who have palpitations, chest pain, and anxiety when the doctor can find no other cause. Once given an inaccurate diagnosis, the patient goes through life treating a cardiac problem that doesn't exist.

Such was the case of Lila, a high-strung trial lawyer, who suffered severe palpitations and chest pain. She was thin, smoked incessantly, and was a vegetarian. When her family doctor heard a click in her heart, he made a diagnosis of mitral valve prolapse.

Lila was given a beta-blocking drug. Her palpitations lessened and the chest pain receded, but after a few months her energy level diminished. This dynamo had become listless. She lost her interest in sex. Her husband urged her to visit the doctor again. She decided to go to a cardiologist for a second opinion.

The cardiologist agreed that she had a click, but the echocardiogram revealed no prolapse. The cardiologist also confirmed she did not suffer from coronary artery disease. The doctor told Lila to discontinue her medication, quit smoking, and stop drinking five cups of coffee a day. The doctor also prescribed an exercise program for Lila and urged her to take some time off for recreation once a month.

Soon after following his advice, Lila was symptom-free.

TREATING MITRAL VALVE PROLAPSE

When mitral valve prolapse is definitively diagnosed, the patient will need a preventive course of penicillin whenever she receives dental care. This precaution is necessary because bacteria from the mouth can get into the blood and race to the roughened mitral valve, causing endocarditis. To prevent endocarditis, antibiotics also should be taken before any invasive procedure, such as surgery or having tubes placed into any orifice of the body.

As some women become older, a prolapsed valve can deteriorate, become calcified, and leak more profoundly, causing regurgitation of blood backward. When this happens, the condition is called mitral insufficiency. At this point, the valve may need to be replaced through open-heart surgery.

The chest pain that caused the patient to seek medical attention is sometimes difficult to treat. Medical science has not clearly determined why chest pain or palpitations accompany mitral valve prolapse.

I encourage my patients with floppy valve syndrome to enter into a solid, regular exercise program, which often relieves the pain. Also, beta-blocking drugs such as Inderal often can relieve the pain as well as the palpitations.

A CASE STUDY IN FLOPPY VALVE SYNDROME

Prolapse of the mitral valve is a lifetime abnormality, but it need not interfere with a patient's lifestyle. Dorothy's heart murmur, for example, was discovered when she was twenty. For years, she had palpitations that lasted up to an hour. During her pregnancy, her heart raced so badly that the doctors had to give her special medications to keep it under control. For many years after giving birth, however, she was relatively symptom-free.

By the time she reached age seventy, her heart murmur had become louder. Echocardiography was then available to confirm the diagnosis of mitral valve prolapse syndrome. She was told to take antibiotics before dental work, but she needed no treatment beyond that.

She and a group of friends organized a swim club for older women, with whom Dorothy swims a mile every morning. Each year, Dorothy allows my medical students to listen to her heart in order to familiarize them with the telltale sounds of mitral valve prolapse.

CHAPTER 7

PALPITATIONS

Palpitations—among the most common complaints of young women patients in my cardiology practice—manifest differently in different people. For some, palpitations mean a fast heartbeat, or tachycardia. Others describe it as a skipped beat, a slow beat, an irregular beat, a fluttering sensation, or a thumping, throbbing feeling. Several patients have said it feels as if their heart is doing a somersault. Palpitations often cause the sufferer to feel dizzy, light-headed, faint, and as though something terrible is going to happen.

To the cardiologist, palpitations mean a fast regular or irregular beat, or a series of skipped beats (extrasystoles), also called premature ventricular contraction (PVC). These skipped beats may or may not be felt by the patient.

Palpitations can have nothing to do with the heart. Excessive movement of gas through the intestine, for example, can cause fluttering sensations in the chest.

Some thin-chested people become conscious of their

heartbeat in a quiet room. This occurs because the person has too little fat on their chest wall to mute the transmission of heart sounds. They mistakenly interpret the normal "lub-dub" beating as palpitations.

Real palpitations can be diagnosed using an electrocardiogram or Holter monitor. Patients who wear Holter monitors are asked to keep a diary so they can jot down the time and duration of each palpitation episode. The diary entries are compared to the readout from the Holter monitor. If the ECG tracing showed no abnormality when the patient felt the palpitations, the sensation did not arise from the heart. When there is a correlation, the ECG can specify which type of palpitations are afflicting the patient.

SUPRAVENTRICULAR TACHYCARDIA

A very rapid, regular heartbeat is called supraventricular tachycardia. This is a very common condition found more often in young women than in young men. Suddenly feeling your heart race like a runaway train is a frightening sensation. It can drop your blood pressure and make you perspire and feel faint.

CAUSES. In some cases, supraventricular tachycardia is triggered by excessive caffeine intake, smoking, severe anxiety, medications such as antihistamines or asthma drugs, an overactive thyroid gland, cocaine, alcohol, mitral valve prolapse (see Chapter 6), or congenital electrical conduction abnormalities. Most of the time, however, doctors are unable to pinpoint a cause for supraventricular tachycardia.

If the cause or causes can be identified and eliminated, the tachycardia may disappear.

TREATMENTS. If you have a fast heartbeat that does not subside on its own, you may be a candidate for a new medication called adenosine, which stops the tachycardia in minutes. It is commonly administered in the emergency room. Other medications used to prevent supraventricular tachycardia include digoxin, beta-blockers, and channel blockers.

There also are nonmedicinal treatments to curb rapid heartbeats. I taught my daughters, both of whom suffer from this condition, to start coughing rapidly as soon as they feel a skipped beat, which often triggers supraventricular tachycardia. I find this method to be the best and safest way to terminate the attack.

Other methods include:

- Making yourself gag by putting your finger in back of the throat
- Bearing down as if for a bowel movement
- Squatting and bearing down
- Rapidly drinking a glass of cold water
- Singing loudly
- Massaging your carotid artery (located on either side of the neck)

It's important to consult your doctor before trying any of these techniques.

ATRIAL FIBRILLATION

Atrial fibrillation is an irregular heartbeat that occurs when the upper chamber of the heart (the atrium) twitches and vibrates like a bag of worms. This causes the heart to beat erratically instead of contracting evenly.

Atrial fibrillation made the evening news when former

President George Bush fell victim to it because of an overactive thyroid condition called hyperthyroidism. Mother Teresa suffers from atrial fibrillation. So did Gustav Mahler, the famous Viennese composer. When Mahler heard his own heart beating erratically, he wrote a symphony to it.

Galen, the young Greek doctor of the second century A.D., worked as a physician for the gladiators. Once when a gladiator was mortally wounded, his chest split wide open. Galen removed the beating heart, which was fibrillating. As he ran through the arena with the heart in his hand, the cheering crowd witnessed the heart twitching and beating on its own. This grisly demonstration proved that the heart has its own electrical power, pacemaker, and conduction system, all of which spread the impulses in an orderly fashion from the top chambers to the bottom to make the heart contract. Atrial fibrillation occurs when the electrical system acts abnormally.

Atrial fibrillation afflicts 5 to 10 percent of people over age sixty and as many as 20 percent of the seventy-and-older population. More than half of atrial fibrillation sufferers are women.

Some patients have slow fibrillation, which may cause no symptoms. Rapid fibrillation can make a person lightheaded and weak and cause shortness of breath. By the time medical attention is sought, the fibrillation may have terminated spontaneously.

CAUSES. Atrial fibrillation can be caused by long-standing hypertension or a blockage of coronary arteries. Rheumatic heart disease, caused by rheumatic fever, was once the most common cause of atrial fibrillation. Rheumatic fever has become uncommon in the United States thanks to penicillin's ability to cure streptococcal infections, which cause rheumatic fever. In older persons atrial fibrillation may be caused by a degeneration of the conduction system of the heart. In some cases of atrial fibrillation, no cause can be found.

DIAGNOSIS. An ECG or Holter monitoring can usually detect atrial fibrillation. Some people whose only complaint is palpitations or anxiety attacks go on for years without their atrial fibrillation being discovered.

TREATMENTS. Sometimes atrial fibrillation reverts back to a normal rhythm on its own. Most of the time, however, treatment is necessary to convert the atrial fibrillation to a normal rhythm, or to keep the pulse rate within an acceptable range. One form of treatment is called cardioversion, where the patient is given an electrical shock to bring the heart rhythm back to normal. Drugs also can be used to normalize the heartbeat.

Sometimes, in spite of all our efforts, atrial fibrillation persists. Our goal then becomes to keep the pulse down to an acceptable rate.

The drug of choice for atrial fibrillation is digoxin, which slows the heart rate. Along with digoxin, the cardiologist may also prescribe procainamide and some newer drugs.

Despite the multiple medications available to treat rapid atrial fibrillation, at times the condition can be extraordinarily difficult to control. And the drugs used can themselves be dangerous, as one of my patients, Patricia, found out.

For a number of years after her last pregnancy, Patricia complained of palpitations, fainting spells, and weakness. She underwent dozens of ECGs, Holter monitorings, and exercise stress tests, but doctors were unable to document any fast or irregular heartbeats. Patricia became seriously depressed. She decided to see a psychiatrist because everyone began doubting that anything was wrong with her heart. Even Patricia began to wonder if she was imagining all those weird sensations in her chest.

One night, her boyfriend, a medical student, placed his ear on her naked chest and was startled to hear her heart racing, like a wildly beating drum. Finally, Patricia had confirmation that something was wrong.

During her first appointment with me, Patricia's heart suddenly started to race as I was examining her. We performed an ECG immediately. The test disclosed that Patricia was suffering from very rapid atrial fibrillation. Her heart rate would jump to more than 200 beats per minute, almost triple the normal rate. It was a fortuitous finding on my part, as it had been with her boyfriend.

Unable to trace the cause of her condition, I put Patricia on medication. But the drug not only failed to control her atrial fibrillation, it produced nausea and other, more severe side effects.

Finally, I put her in the hospital where she was given a new test for racing hearts called electrophysiological testing. This test measures the way the electrical circuits of the heart are working. The test showed that my patient would benefit most from a new treatment for this type of tachycardia called catheter ablation therapy. During the therapy, radio frequency waves are used to destroy the heart's abnormal conduction tract, thus curing the atrial fibrillation.

Most people with atrial fibrillation can engage in everyday activities, including exercise, so long as it's under the guidance of a cardiologist.

There is a darker side to this disorder. During fibrillation, clots form in the chambers of the heart. These clots can break off and can travel to the brain, causing a stroke, or to other arteries of the body. Because of this clotting action, atrial fibrillation is responsible for about 75,000 strokes each year. More than half of these strokes could have been prevented with blood-thinning drugs.

The first blood-thinner, also known as an anticoagulant, was discovered in the early 1920s when a strange cattle disease broke out in North Dakota and Alberta, Canada. The cattle were bleeding to death because they ate hay prepared from spoiled clover. The chemical that caused the bleeding was discovered in the clover and named dicumarol.

For a long time, the effectiveness of dicumarol and related drugs was highly controversial. It took many years of medical trials to show that dicumarol (sold as Coumadin) and other blood-thinners, taken in low dosages, can prevent clotting in humans. One of those studies was conducted by Dr. Michael Ezekowitz at the Yale Medical School, who demonstrated that blood-thinners could prevent strokes. Aspirin also was tested but was found not to be as effective as Coumadin in preventing strokes in patients suffering from atrial fibrillation.

Dicumarol, which was initially used as rat poison, has become the primary drug used to prevent blood clots in patients with atrial fibrillation, phlebitis (inflammation of a vein), and pulmonary embolism. Despite its usefulness, at this writing, Coumadin is not being prescribed for most people suffering from long-standing atrial fibrillation. If you are suffering from atrial fibrillation, consider asking your doctor about Coumadin. Adults of any age can take it, although it is not recommended for pregnant women.

Patients must be careful when taking Coumadin because it can cause serious hemorrhage in the brain and intestines. The dosage has to be scrupulously monitored by the doctor or the blood can become too thin, which results in hemorrhages. The dosage is determined by a frequent blood test, called the prothrombin time test.

Patients taking Coumadin or any anticoagulant are cautioned not too take many aspirins because hemorrhage can result. Other medications, such as phenobarbital, can double Coumadin's blood-thinning effect and cause hemorrhage. Serious trauma to the head and body also can result in hemorrhage in patients taking anticoagulants. Prior to dental extraction or any surgery, Coumadin must be discontinued for at least three days.

Another anticoagulant we now use to prevent strokes and pulmonary embolism is called heparin. Discovered by a premed student in 1922, heparin also is used during the early hours of a heart attack to help prevent further clotting in the coronary arteries.

SKIPPED BEATS AND MISSED BEATS

Skipped beats (extrasystoles), missed beats, or premature beats are very common and have many potential causes. It is prudent to suspect one of these problems if your palpitations actually feel like your heart is skipping or missing a beat.

CAUSES. The most typical causes are too much alcohol, cigarette smoking, anxiety, or a diseased heart muscle.

Skipped beats are very common when the heart is damaged from alcohol (cardiomyopathy), or after a heart attack. These skipped beats are not usually dangerous unless they are associated with an abnormal heart muscle. Many patients suffer from skipped beats all their lives. If there are no other cardiac abnormalities, it is best not to treat skipped beats, except to eliminate caffeine, cigarettes, and alcohol. Exercise and stress-reduction programs can further reduce extrasystoles.

Skipped beats or premature contractions in the presence of a heart attack, or in patients suffering from cardiomyopathy, require antiarrhythmic medications because these irregular heartbeats can lead to sudden death. At one time, physicians were rather liberal in the administration of medications to eliminate extrasystoles. Then several studies showed that the death rate can be worse with these drugs than without them.

To reduce the risk of serious side effects or sudden death, antiarrythmics must be administered by doctors who are well versed in the use of these drugs. Treating abnormal heart rhythms has become so complicated that it has given rise to a new branch of cardiology called electrophysiology. Electrophysiology specialists are experts in the administration of such drugs as amiodarone, sotalol, digoxin, disopyramide, flecainide, propafenone, lidocaine, mexiletine, procainamide, quinidine, and tocainide.

HEART BLOCK

When the heart rate slows to below 60 beats per minute, it is called bradycardia. Bradycardia can be present but harmless in healthy athletes because their hearts are highly conditioned. If the heart rate drops to 40 or 30 beats per minute in nonathletic older people, however, it could mean the heart's electrical system is blocked and is failing to conduct impulses all the way through the heart muscle. This so-called complete heart block may result from clogged arteries and an aging heart, although certain medications, such as digoxin, and low potassium levels in the blood can be to blame.

SYMPTOMS. In the older woman, bradycardia can lead to the brain receiving too little blood because the heart is pumping too slowly. When this happens, the symptoms can include fainting, dizzy spells, weakness, memory loss, disorientation, and confusion. Ironically, bradycardia also can produce a sensation of palpitations in some patients.

TREATMENT. Many people with a slow heart rate suffer no symptoms and need no treatment. When bradycardia produces symptoms, the treatment is a pacemaker.

There are different kinds of pacemakers, but all work on the same principle. The pacemaker automatically emits a pulse of electricity, which keeps the heart rate from dipping below 50 beats per minute.

Small and compact, the pacemaker is barely visible after it is implanted under the skin of the chest wall. Once the pacemaker is implanted, the fainting, dizzy spells and weakness caused by inadequate blood flow subside.

There are more than 2.5 million pacemaker users in the United States, and most are women. The average pacemaker user is over age seventy. Pacemakers have been shown to prolong life of both men and women by at least twelve years.

VENTRICULAR TACHYCARDIA

Ventricular tachycardia is a serious type of abnormally fast heart rhythm that is responsible for palpitations. It usually results from coronary artery disease and enlarged hearts, but it also can stem from a heart attack or cardiomyopathy. In ventricular tachycardia, the heart races to 140 to 220 beats per minute. The condition can cause victims to collapse and sometimes leads to cardiac arrest (heart stops beating). Patients who arrive in the emergency room with ventricular tachycardia often have to be electrically shocked to break the abnormal rhythm and convert it to normal (cardioversion).

Patients with recurrent ventricular tachycardia that cannot be controlled with medications can have a device called an automatic implantable cardioverter-defibrillator system (AICD) implanted into their hearts to convert the irregular rhythm to normal.

I recall one unusual case of a patient named Jane, who underwent a sex-change operation at Yale New Haven Hospital. Jane became James, a robust man who smoked and took male hormones weekly.

Several years after the operation, James suffered several heart attacks and needed a bypass operation, which was successful. But his heart had been damaged, and James had recurrent episodes of ventricular tachycardia. In an effort to cure his potentially fatal disorder, James had another sex-change operation and became Jane again. For this, he had to take estrogen, a female hormone. But Jane continued to have the life-threatening abnormal heart rhythms.

Jane became one of the first people to receive AICD. Each time her heart launched into this dangerous rhythm, the AICD shocked her, putting her entire body into a spasm for a few seconds. The process took some getting used to, but a year later, Jane was doing well with her defibrillator. She no longer smoked or took estrogen. She looked like her old self again, and had even taken a male lover.

Another miracle of medicine.

CHAPTER 8

VASCULAR DISEASE

Just as coronary arteries can suffer the ravages of cholesterol-caked blockages, the arteries of the legs, abdomen, and head also can fall prey. Smoking, a major cause of hardening of the coronary arteries, contributes to blockages of other arteries in the body. Obesity, high cholesterol, diabetes, and hypertension are other factors that can aggravate vascular disease.

This chapter will explore the three most common forms of noncardiac vascular disease that afflict women:

- Peripheral vascular disease (PVD)—a blockage in the arteries of the legs;
- Aneurysms—swelling of an artery in the abdomen or chest; and
- Carotid artery disease—a blockage in one or more of the four main arteries in the neck and head.

PERIPHERAL VASCULAR DISEASE (PVD)

In 1992, an extensive ten-year study reported that 20 percent of women over age sixty had peripheral vascular disease, or PVD—a blockage in the arteries of the lower extremities. A high percentage of women with PVD also had silent coronary artery disease—severe blockages of the coronary arteries with no symptoms. The study further found that the women with PVD had a three to fifteen times greater risk of premature death than women without PVD. Any woman diagnosed with PVD, therefore, should be given a thallium stress test (see Chapter 5) because she is at high risk for coronary artery disease.

DIAGNOSING PVD. In order to diagnose peripheral vascular disease, the doctor uses a stethoscope to check the pulses of the neck (carotid arteries), the belly (abdominal aorta), the top of the thigh (femoral arteries), the crease behind the knee (popliteal artery), the top of the foot (pedial artery), and just below the ankle bone (posterior tibial artery). If the pulses in any of these arteries are diminished or absent, peripheral vascular disease is probably the cause.

SYMPTOMS. Eighty percent of people with PVD have no symptoms of the disease. The other 20 percent experience the classic symptoms: pain or cramps in the thigh, calves, or just above the ankles, depending upon where the blockage is located. The pain first becomes evident after walking and is relieved during rest. As the blockage worsens, the leg pain begins to persist, even when walking is discontinued. Soon, the woman may walk comfortably—until the pain strikes again, much as angina pain comes and goes.

The pain is triggered when the leg muscle becomes

starved for oxygen because an artery is obstructed. As the artery becomes almost totally blocked, the feet may tingle or feel cold and numb. These sensations may or may not be accompanied by pain. The feet become pale, like a cadaver's. In about 5 percent of cases, usually in women diabetics who delayed their care, the toes turn a trifle blue, later becoming as blue-green as the Caribbean. At this late stage, a vascular surgeon may be able to perform a bypass operation on the artery to save the leg. In some cases, amputation is the only solution.

Fortunately, peripheral vascular disease can be prevented and possibly reversed, as in the case of one of my patients, Helga.

Helga was always envied by her friends because she is thin, beautiful, and successful. Despite the fact that she smoked, Helga was a terrific tennis player, an accomplished downhill skier, and she competed in equestrian contests every year. For years, her husband begged her to give up smoking.

The first sign that something was wrong with Helga occurred while she was vacationing in Paris, strolling on the Champs-Elysées. She suddenly developed cramps in both calves. The cramps subsided, and she told no one about the incident. She felt fine for several months until one day, while playing tennis, she felt a terrible burning in both of her ankles. The pain was so excruciating that she had to quit the match.

The burning pain came back each time she played tennis, usually striking about ten minutes after the second game. Helga made her own diagnosis of inflamed tendons and visited a podiatrist, who on two occasions injected both feet with cortisone. He gave her five ultrasound treatments, whirlpool therapy, and supports for her shoes.

Helga's pain became worse, which baffled the podiatrist. Another shot of cortisone? Different supports for her shoes? He wasn't sure how to proceed.

Fortunately, Helga was not only intelligent, but reasonably honest with herself. She went to see her internist, who knew she smoked too much. The pulses in her legs were a little weak, so the internist performed some vascular exams, including one using Doppler imaging, which measures the flow of blood through the vessels.

The internist discovered that after strenuous exercise the flow through Helga's leg arteries decreased dramatically. The blood pressure in her calves dropped below that in her arms. The doctor then performed ultrasound and Doppler exams of the arteries and found that the arteries in Helga's lower legs were blocked.

That discovery prompted Helga to finally quit smoking. She was put on Trental, a medication that improves blood flow, and one aspirin daily. Despite relatively good eating habits, her cholesterol was elevated, so she also was placed on a strict low-fat diet.

After six months, Helga's condition improved. She could play tennis pain-free. One year later, vascular exams showed a marked improvement in the flow of blood, and her exercise stress test was normal. Three hundred dollars' worth of shoe inlays sit in her closet, a reminder that a correct diagnosis is the first step to getting well.

Another patient, Carrie, illustrates a different clinical picture of peripheral vascular disease. Carrie is an overweight diabetic who does not smoke and leads a full and active life as a hospital secretary. She is a single parent who regulates her own insulin dosage and feels well most of the time, except for fatigue at the end of an especially busy day.

At her last routine medical exam, the doctor, as a matter of course, checked the pulses in her legs and found them to be diminished. Carrie always gave scrupulous care to her feet, inspecting them daily for ulcers, calluses, and corns, and she wore sensible shoes. Despite her precautions, she noticed that her feet seemed pale. She had no leg pain or cramps. Nonetheless, a Doppler examination showed severe closure of both arteries of the lower legs. Diabetics often have a blunted response to pain, which may explain Carrie's lack of symptoms.

Her doctor ordered a magnetic resonance imaging test, which confirmed that her leg arteries were severely blocked. An X ray of the arteries (angiogram) showed that very little blood was able to pass through.

Because Carrie was at risk for heart disease, she took a thallium stress test, which was very abnormal. A cardiac catheterization showed that all three of her coronary arteries were blocked.

Carrie's legs were saved with balloon angioplasty (see Chapter 14). Regarding her blocked coronary arteries, all the specialists who examined Carrie agreed that it would be too dangerous to wait to reverse her atherosclerosis through diet and medications, even though she had no symptoms of coronary artery disease.

After the angioplasty on her legs, Carrie underwent a successful coronary bypass operation. She now follows a program of weight reduction and leg exercises designed to prevent a recurrence of blocked arteries.

EXERCISE. The leg exercises recommended for patients prone to peripheral vascular disease are simple and effective. The patient simply rises up on her toes as many times as she can. At first, many women with PVD cannot do more than twenty repetitions. Gradually, though, many are able to build up to one hundred.

In most cases, prevention programs like Carrie's effectively combat PVD because the exercises lead to the formation of "collateral blood vessels"—new channels for blood to nourish the legs—and the special diet decreases artery-clogging cholesterol plaques.

ANEURYSMS

When the wall of an artery becomes weakened and swells like a balloon, it is called an aneurysm. If an aneurysm forms in the chest, the condition is known as a thoracic aortic aneurysm; if in the abdomen, it is called an abdominal aortic aneurysm. As the ballooned wall increases in size, it stretches thinner and thinner and can suddenly, without the slightest warning, burst and result in a fatal hemorrhage.

Sometimes a thoracic aortic aneurysm can be seen on a chest X ray. In the case of an abdominal aneurysm, a doctor can sometimes feel it in the abdomen of a female patient who is thin. In heavy people, it is almost impossible to feel an abdominal aneurysm unless it has become extremely large. In most cases, it is very difficult to diagnose an aneurysm because there are very few symptoms.

Symptoms, when they are present, can manifest in back pain if the aorta pushes to the rear as it enlarges. I recommend that women who have a family history of a burst (ruptured) aneurysm have an ultrasound examination of the abdomen at least once after menopause. I also advise abdominal ultrasound for women over age sixty who smoke cigarettes or have any of the following conditions:

- Diabetes
- Hypertension
- Peripheral vascular disease
- Obesity
- Coronary artery disease
- Excessive fats in the blood
- New back pain

If a small abdominal aneurysm is found, it can be followed up by periodic ultrasound examinations. If it begins to enlarge, the only treatment is surgery. A rupture of an aneurysm and death can be avoided if the woman knows in advance that she is at risk for such an event. Once the aneurysm ruptures, the chances of survival are poor unless the rupture is swiftly discovered and a surgical team is on hand to operate immediately.

CAROTID ARTERY DISEASE

In the neck, there are two primary arteries (right and left carotid arteries) that each divide into two main branches (internal and external). Just like coronary arteries, carotid arteries can become narrowed or blocked by cholesterol plaques. To diagnose a plaque build-up in these important vessels, the doctor uses a stethoscope to listen to the blood flowing through. If the doctor hears a swishing sound known as a bruit, it could indicate that a cholesterol plaque is blocking one of the carotid arteries.

Any woman diagnosed with coronary artery disease, peripheral vascular disease, or an abdominal aneurysm should undergo tests to see whether the carotid arteries are blocked. Ultrasound and Doppler examinations can show the extent of any blockages that may exist.

It is estimated that even patients with no symptoms have a 5 percent risk each year for stroke stemming from a blocked carotid artery. Because the blockage cuts off the blood supply to the brain, a temporary or permanent paralysis of the legs or arms can follow. Paralysis sometimes is accompanied by loss of vision and the inability to speak, which also may be temporary or permanent.

SURGERY. A severely narrowed carotid artery can be opened during a delicate operation called an endarterectomy. While an endarterectomy can restore normal blood flow to the brain by removing the fatty plaque buildup, there is controversy over whether to operate on blocked carotid arteries if the patient has no symptoms. The reason is the risk. Some patients suffer a permanent stroke during the surgery. And many patients live a normal life span without surgery, despite the blockage. As with all surgeries, success of the endarterectomy depends on the experience of the surgeon. Newer techniques are being developed that will make the surgery safer and more effective.

MEDICATION. Aspirin has been shown to be effective in preventing strokes, even among patients with carotid artery disease. I recommend that all women at risk for stroke take one baby aspirin a day. A new drug called Ticlid (Ticlopidine) is also used for prevention of strokes.

Women who have carotid artery disease are prone to have little strokes, or transient ischemic attacks (TIA). TIAs produce symptoms that appear and disappear within twenty-four hours. These include any of the following:

- Blurred vision or loss of vision
- Dizziness
- Weakness or numbness of the face
- Loss of speech
- Change in personality

If you have suffered a TIA, you should undergo thorough neurological and cardiac examinations in order to evaluate your risks for a full-blown stroke or coronary artery disease. You may require hospitalization to thin out your blood with heparin to try to prevent a full blown stroke.

CHAPTER 9

VARICOSE VEINS

As in other veins, the veins of the legs have valves that keep the blood traveling in one direction—toward the heart. If the valves become damaged or are inherently weak, the blood will stagnate and pool in the area. This stagnation causes the ankles or the entire leg to swell, damaging the walls of the veins. Eventually, the swelling leads to the veins in the legs becoming torturous and swollen, a condition commonly known as varicose veins. Hippocrates first described varicose veins 2,500 years ago. Today, as many as one in five women have the condition.

Faulty valves are only one reason blood can pool in the legs. Obesity, pregnancy, straining during bowel movements, and tumors in the abdomen also can put pressure on veins and block the return of blood to the heart. In some women, varicose veins make their debut during pregnancy and never go away. Prolonged sitting, excessive retention of fluids, and medications such as calcium channel blockers can cause the ankles to swell. Swollen ankles also may be a symptom of heart disease or kidney failure.

Most people regard varicose veins as unsightly. But cosmetic concerns pale when compared to the potential health problems this condition can cause. If neglected, varicose veins can grow as large as grapes and become a site for inflammation (phlebitis), blood clots (thrombosis), or both conditions simultaneously—thrombophlebitis. Each year, up to 2 million women develop phlebitis and clots, and many also have varicose veins. A clot can break off and travel to the lungs, creating a life-threatening condition called a pulmonary embolism (see Chapter 10).

SYMPTOMS. The most noticeable symptom of varicose veins is swelling of the ankles and legs. Blue vessels, or "spiders," of the skin along the inner parts of the thighs or elsewhere are not to be confused with varicose veins. Spider veins can be improved by a therapy involving the injection of chemicals.

Significant varicose veins can cause such symptoms as a nagging feeling in the legs and fatigue, especially at the end of the day when ankle swelling is at its worst. If the veins become inflamed, red, and swollen, the patient will suffer a great deal of pain in her leg or ankle.

Discomfort in the calf can emerge after a minor injury to the leg, a long car or plane trip, or even being immobilized in the hospital. The discomfort may soon be followed by a seemingly trivial red spot over the varicose vein site, which may enlarge like a rising sun.

The patient may find that her leg pain is relieved when she lies flat. But the pain returns when she stands up because blood again expands the walls of the veins.

PREVENTION. Proper care of varicose veins can prevent phlebitis and clots. First, avoid cigarettes. Smoking accelerates clot formation in the veins and arteries. Second, be extra careful to avoid injuring the areas affected by varicose veins. Even a minor injury to a varicose vein can sometimes cause an ulcer. This condition is very difficult to treat and requires prolonged management by a doctor who specializes in varicose vein care.

During long car, rail, or airplane trips, wear good-quality elastic stockings, which help prevent the stagnation of blood in the varicose veins. Also during long trips, stand up and walk around once an hour or whenever possible. During these breaks, lift yourself up on your toes fifty times (or as many times as you can). Exercise is an excellent way to prevent clots and phlebitis because it keeps the blood flowing and helps prevent the platelets from sticking to one other. Platelet aggravation is one of the important causes of thrombosis.

Another way to make the platelets less sticky is to take one simple aspirin a day, but ask your doctor first.

TREATMENT. Most women who undergo treatment for varicose veins do so for cosmetic reasons, but medical reasons are much more compelling.

Many patients benefit from sclerotherapy, injections of a special solution into the varicose veins in order to collapse them. The Mayo Clinic popularized sclerotherapy sixty years ago. Recently, there has been renewed interest in managing varicose veins with sclerotherapy, even when the treatment has to be repeated every two years or more frequently.

If injections or other medical treatments fail, or your doctor does not think sclerotherapy will help, surgery may be needed to remove the varicose veins. The benefits of surgery last longer, but like sclerotherapy, surgery may have to be repeated if varicose veins return.

Inflammation of varicose veins is called superficial phlebitis. Treatment for superficial phlebitis consists of bed rest, elevating the legs, warm soaks, antibiotics, and anti-inflammatory drugs. Most patients who follow this regimen achieve pain relief in a few days, but a few weeks of treatment is usually needed to make the swelling and pain go away.

If an ultrasound shows clots in the deep veins, patients usually are given blood-thinners such as heparin or Coumadin or other blood clot busters. In the near future, leech products (hirudin) may also be used (see Chapter 4).

CHAPTER 10

PULMONARY EMBOLISM

Pulmonary embolism means that a clot has traveled to the lungs and has blocked off the pulmonary arteries. This can be fatal. In fact, pulmonary embolism is responsible for one third of all sudden deaths in the United States. It can happen to anyone of any age at any time. Yet, this catastrophic condition doesn't get near the attention given to AIDS, heart attacks, or cancer.

The major cause of pulmonary embolism are clots in the deep veins and thrombophlebitis (see Chapter 9). A pulmonary embolism also can result from surgery, a malignancy, pregnancy, or clots in the heart chamber. Obesity, birth control pills, heart failure, and lung disease are considered risk factors. Sometimes the origin of the embolism is not found.

Each year in the United States, there are about 500,000 pulmonary embolisms, which kill some 160,000 Americans. I believe we could cut the death rate from massive pulmonary embolism in half if women were aware that it can occur and reminded their doctors that it is always a possibility. Being assertive, especially if you are at risk for a pulmonary embolism, is an important way to take charge of your own body and become a partner in your medical care.

SYMPTOMS. One reason pulmonary embolisms are so deadly is that they frequently go undiagnosed and are often confused with a heart attack because both conditions can cause chest pain. The main reason pulmonary embolism is frequently misdiagnosed in women is because its symptoms may be dismissed as anxiety, hyperventilation, hysteria, or depression.

Some of the symptoms of a pulmonary embolism are severe anxiety and shortness of breath, usually accompanied by chest pain. (Anytime a woman experiences chest pain, she should seek medical attention right away.) A woman who has symptoms of a potential pulmonary embolism should undergo a diagnostic test called a lung scan. Sometimes it is necessary to confirm the results of the lung scan with an angiogram of the pulmonary artery. A dye is injected through a catheter and X rays are taken of the pulmonary artery to see if it is blocked by a clot. Another test that helps in the diagnosis is a ventilation test, which shows whether the distribution of blood in the lungs is normal.

TREATMENT. Once a pulmonary embolism is diagnosed, the patient usually receives an anticoagulant such as heparin intravenously for up to ten days, and then takes the oral anticoagulant Coumadin for about six months to a year.

CASE STUDIES OF PULMONARY EMBOLISM

Leslie was thirty-eight years old and on her second career. She smoked incessantly and had been on birth control pills for three months after she became romantically involved with a much younger man.

Their relationship ended abruptly, leaving Leslie distraught. She began having panic attacks in the morning. Sometimes in the late afternoon, she'd begin hyperventilating. Her doctor told her to breathe into a paper bag to depress the respiratory center whenever she hyperventilated. It helped.

While at work one December afternoon, Leslie started to breathe rapidly, feel faint, and experience some chest pain. She ran into the bathroom, placed her brown lunch bag on her face and breathed her own breath. But this time, her symptoms persisted. Her heart was racing, and she felt increasingly faint. Her supervisor rushed her to the emergency room of a nearby hospital.

Her ECG was slightly abnormal, and the doctor on duty, a young intern, ordered a chest X ray, which was normal. The amount of oxygen in her blood was slightly decreased. She was given a tranquilizer and soon felt well enough to return to work. That night, she was brought back to the emergency room wheezing badly. She was told she had asthma and given medication for it. Two hours later, she died suddenly at the hospital. An autopsy showed a massive embolism in both lungs, and clots in the veins of her legs.

It's possible that Leslie would have survived if she had told the emergency room physicians that she smoked and took oral contraceptives. The older birth control pills can cause clots to form, especially in women who smoke. The new contraceptive pills contain a lower dose of hormones and are less likely to cause an embolism.

Betty, forty-nine, spent five days traveling up the Nile. The food made her so ill that she never left the boat to see the ruins at Luxor. She stayed in bed, close to the toilet. Soon afterward, she spent ten miserable hours on a plane.

Two days after returning home, Betty developed a dry cough, and her chest hurt each time she took a deep breath. She went to her doctor, who admitted her to the hospital. A chest X ray showed a shadow, which the doctors decided was pneumonia.

Two days of antibiotics did not help. Betty's condition grew worse. Her temperature climbed, and her chest pain became more frequent and intense.

A lung scan showed that her lungs were showered with clots from an embolism. An ultrasound examination of her thighs disclosed that numerous clots in her femoral vein had broken through and traveled to her lungs. After ten days of thinning out her blood with heparin, Betty's symptoms subsided. Her life was saved.

Selma, a two-pack-a-day smoker, had a face that looked like a road map. She was once told that smoking cigarettes causes wrinkles. She saw a plastic surgeon, who agreed to perform a face-lift. A few days after her surgery, while still in the hospital, Selma became anxious and frightened as she wondered what explanation to give her friends for her new "self." Her anxiety led to hyperventilation. Selma then became aware of "a funny feeling" in her chest.

The nurse on call that night was smart enough to notify her internist instead of giving Selma the tranquilizer that had been prescribed for her. The internist immediately ordered a lung scan, which was very abnormal. More tests followed, and there was no doubt that Selma had sustained a pulmonary embolism.

She was treated with an anticoagulant and survived. She gave up smoking. The lines on her face seem less important to her now than they once did.

PART II

PREVENTION AND TREATMENT OF HEART DISEASE IN WOMEN

CHAPTER 11

DIET AND MEDICATIONS FOR PREVENTING HEART ATTACK

By this point in the book, you should realize that heart disease does not appear overnight and heart attacks are not isolated events. These problems are, in almost all cases, in the making for decades before symptoms appear.

With the cornucopia of drugs and legion of high-tech medical treatments currently available, it's easy to assume the miracles of modern medicine will be there when you need them in an emergency situation. While medical science is able to prolong tens of thousands of lives every year, heart disease remains the number one killer of Americans. It is clear, therefore, that no matter how sophisticated a test or treatment is, nothing is as effective as preventive medicine.

As pointed out in the first part of this book, quitting smoking is one of the most important steps you can take to improve your heart and overall health. I will not belabor the tobacco issue here. This chapter will discuss other things you can do to prevent a heart attack, including lowering your cholesterol, losing weight, and taking certain medications to improve your cardiovascular system.

CONTROLLING CHOLESTEROL WITH DIET

That diets rich in fat cause early death is an old story. Nicholas II, the last czar of Russia (who was assassinated in 1917), was chagrined that members of his pampered elite honor guard had short life spans while the poor peasants, with their simple diet of grains and vegetables, lived longer.

In 1908, Dr. A. I. Ignatowski of St. Petersburg hypothesized that the elite guardsmen were dying prematurely because of their diets, which were rich in meats and salty caviar. Dr. Ignatowski fed rabbits with the sumptuous meals typical of the czar's court and saw that the animals developed hardening of the arteries. When Ignatowski's experiments were repeated by other scientists on monkeys and dogs, the same atherosclerosis plaques were found.

During World War II, the Germans stole all the cows from the Scandinavian countries. When the Scandinavians' consumption of milk and meat dropped drastically—so did their heart attack rates. After the war, the cows—and the heart attacks—were back.

In 1958, Dr. William Dock, a highly skilled and visionary cardiologist, told a group of physicians gathered for a meeting in Atlantic City, New Jersey, that coronary artery disease is a reversible illness. While his assertion was on target, there was little hard evidence showing that people who cut down their fat intake lived longer. Not surprisingly, the physicians in Dock's audience greeted his optimistic view with skepticism.

Since then, the link between a high-fat diet and heart disease has been confirmed again and again through research studies. In one recent example, researchers found that people from eastern Finland, who consume large amounts of milk and cheese, have the highest average cholesterol counts in the world and the highest rate of coronary heart disease. By contrast, the Japanese in the southern islands eat mostly rice and fish and have some of the world's lowest heart-attack rates.

Despite the preponderance of this evidence, many physicians are still skeptical that fatty plaques can be shrunk through proper diet and medication.

HOW CHOLESTEROL AFFECTS THE HEART. Plaques that form on the inner wall of the arteries are made up of cholesterol (a type of fat), fibrous tissue, and calcium. Generally speaking, this build-up is known as atherosclerosis. This is a further complication of arteriosclerosis, the hardening of the arteries that affects all human beings over time—the arteries lose their elasticity and become firmer as we age. Atherosclerosis is arteriosclerosis plus the build-up of plaque. Unless diet modifications and other changes are made, more plaque buildup can occur, creating a nest for a clot to form.

A blood clot can develop anytime the plaque ruptures and ulcerates. Clotting is the body's natural way of sealing an injured artery. When it happens in a narrowed artery of the heart, a heart attack often ensues.

WHO SHOULD WATCH THEIR FAT INTAKE? Five percent of the population have a genetically high cholesterol level in their blood that is not related to their diet. No matter how much cholesterol and other fats they cut from their diet (saturated fat is notorious for raising the bad LDL cholesterol), their cholesterol count will remain high unless drugs can lower it.

The rest of the population can exert some control over their blood cholesterol level. Anyone with a cholesterol level above 200 should make sure they are not getting more than 300 mg of cholesterol a day. A good target number for your cholesterol level is 180 mg. LDL levels above 160 should prompt fat-cutting dietary changes, as should HDL levels below 35 (see Chapter 3).

Some women (and men) have a cholesterol level as high as 260. But they need not be as vigilant about their fat intake if they have no heart disease, are nonsmokers, have normal blood pressure, are not overweight, and their LDL is normal and HDL is over 60. According to the Framingham Heart Study, which included women, high cholesterol levels did not raise the incidence of heart attacks if the HDL was elevated in women over age fifty.

HOW TO REDUCE FAT. The new food labels mandated by the Food and Drug Administration make it easier to follow a low-fat diet since the amount of fat and percentage of calories derived from fat are clearly stated on virtually all processed-food containers.

One way to reduce fat without leaving yourself hungry is by increasing your intake of complex carbohydrates such as those found in grains, soybeans, pasta, cereals, and popcorn (without butter, of course). Many people have been led to believe that oat bran and other sources of dietary fiber bind with cholesterol and pull it out of the body. But research data thus far has not been very convincing.

The American Heart Association recommends that daily cholesterol intake not exceed 300 mg. Most Americans have a long way to go. The average American diet contains about 800 to 1,000 milligrams of cholesterol each day. With 300 mg of cholesterol packed into a single egg yolk and as much as 600 mg of cholesterol in a six-inch untrimmed steak, it's not difficult to see how easily a person can consume 1,000 mg a day.

With regards to fat, there are dozens of dietary recommendations. I have adapted the following for the average healthy woman: Total fat intake should not exceed 35 percent—10 percent saturated, 15 percent monosaturated, and no more than 10 percent unsaturated fats. (See discussion later in this chapter.)

Logic would dictate that the French—who are famous for their delicious cheeses, pâté, and sinfully rich sauces—would have a high rate of heart attacks. But quite the opposite is true. French cardiologists have supplied evidence that their country's comparatively low heart-attack death rate can be attributed to a lifelong daily intake of red wine. French doctors have claimed that there is some chemical in the wine that offsets the bad effects of cholesterol. Studies into the relationship between red wine and cholesterol are ongoing.

WEIGHT REDUCTION. If you lower your fat intake, chances are you'll also lose weight, an important step toward lowering your risk of heart disease. Losing weight is especially important if you are obese, defined as being 20 to 30 percent or more over your ideal weight.

Although one third of Americans are on a diet at any given time, most fail to keep the weight off on a long-term basis. In fact, 90 percent of dieters regain their lost weight in two years. Millions of people pay billions of dollars each year on commercial diets. Diet vendors make promises but can offer no proof that their method will lead to permanent weight loss. Just ask Oprah Winfrey.

The key to losing weight is coupling your low-fat diet with exercise, the focus of Chapter 18.

CHOLESTEROL-LOWERING MEDICATIONS

Some people, regardless of how hard they try, are unable to bring their cholesterol down to a safe level by losing weight and lowering their fat intake. In these cases, cholesterol-lowering drugs may be helpful. A variety of these drugs have hit the marketplace, and more medications are emerging every year. While these medications are effective, an ideal drug to halt and reverse atherosclerosis has yet to make its debut.

In general, cholesterol-lowering drugs are not recommended unless the patient has failed to lower her cholesterol, LDL, and triglyceride levels through diet after two to six months. Even after she begins taking one or more cholesterol-lowering drugs, the patient must continue to adhere to a low-fat, low-cholesterol diet because the medications alone will not bring the cholesterol to an optimal level.

NIACIN. One of the most popular cholesterol-lowering agents is niacin, a water-soluble B vitamin. Niacin lowers the cholesterol and LDL while raising the HDL. Niacin is actually vitamin B^3—nicotinic acid—which was discovered by Dr. J. Goldberger in 1914 to treat pellagra, a disease that causes nerve damage and turns the skin red and the tongue black.

Niacin was used thirty years ago to combat peripheral vascular disease. Niacin's ability to lower blood cholesterol was discovered during a study called the Coronary Drug Project, which compared different cholesterol-lowering drugs in people who suffered a heart attack in the 1980s. The Coronary Drug Project, performed by the National Institutes of Health throughout the United States in 1986, demonstrated a significant decrease in mortality among men and women who took niacin for fifteen years.

In order to be effective, niacin must be taken in large dosages—1 to 3 grams per day. When taken properly, niacin is the best drug available. It can raise the HDL by

15 to 25 percent and lower the LDL by 10 to 15 percent. It is relatively inexpensive and is sold without a prescription.

Niacin's most annoying side effect is flushing of the face and entire body. It can make you feel like you have a bad sunburn, or that you are experiencing a hot flush. Flushing can last for hours and then subside. Flushing is diminished when niacin is taken in slow-release capsules, or with food or an aspirin. Niacin should not be used by a woman who has stomach ulcers or diabetes because it can aggravate these conditions.

CHOLESTYRAMINE. Cholestyramine (sold under the brand names Questran and Colestid) enhances the body's ability to eliminate cholesterol through the gut. A nationwide study, the Lipid Research Clinics Coronary Prevention Trial, performed by the National Institutes of Health, and completed in the early 1980s, affirmed the effectiveness of cholestyramine in reducing the cholesterol level and decreasing the death rate from heart attacks. People in the study who took cholestyramine had an average decline in blood cholesterol of 25 percent. More importantly,their total heart-attack death rate fell by 49 percent. For each 1 percent drop in cholesterol, there was a 2 percent drop in the death rate.

Cholestyramine works by lowering the LDL by 10 to 30 percent. Even though it reduces bad cholesterol, the drug can sometimes raise the triglyceride level.

Cholestyramine is often poorly tolerated. Its major side effects are constipation and the formation of large amounts of intestinal gas. Cholestyramine also interferes with other drugs, such as digitalis, diuretics, warfarin, fat-soluble vitamins, and beta-blockers. Cholestyramine also can lead to gallstones; therefore women with gallbladder disease should avoid the medication.

Despite the potential adverse effects, cholestyramine is considered the safest of the cholesterol-lowering drugs and has been in use the longest.

Like all the cholesterol-lowering drugs, cholestyramine should be taken in the morning and at bedtime, since the body's production of cholesterol is most active at night.

GEMFIBROZIL. Another cholesterol-lowering drug is gemfibrozil (Lopid), which lowers cholesterol and triglyceride levels in the blood. In one study involving four thousand Finnish men with high cholesterol, gemfibrozil raised the HDL (good cholesterol) by 15 to 20 percent and lowered the LDL (bad cholesterol) by 10 to 15 percent; gemfibrozil also lowered the triglyceride level. The coronary artery disease rate fell by 34 percent among the men studied. Even though women were not included in this study, it's reasonable to say that women also can benefit from gemfibrozil.

The dosage is 600 mg twice a day. Gemfibrozil can be taken in tablet form.

LOVASTATIN. Lovastatin (Mevacor) and Simastatin (Zocar) are the drugs best suited for lowering LDL cholesterol as well as triglycerides. Both can reduce the amount of bad cholesterol by 20 to 40 percent. However, lovastatin can cause liver damage and muscle pain and weakness. Zocar has been shown to reverse coronary artery narrowing.

PROBUCOL. Probucol (Lorelco) can lower LDL by 10 to 15 percent. At the same time, though, it also lowers the HDL, or good cholesterol.

Doctors have expressed renewed interest in this drug because it is a powerful antioxidant. In order for LDL (bad cholesterol) to form plaque on the wall of an artery, it must first undergo a molecular change called oxidation. An antioxidant prevents this molecular change from happening.

COMBINING DRUGS. Frequently, patients with high cholesterol are given a combination of cholesterol-lowering drugs. Women with elevated triglycerides and low HDL whose blood fats fail to go down as a result of diet control and estrogen replacement should take one or more of the aforementioned medications. If the LDL is very high (over 200), I favor trying lovastatin or Simastatin (Zocar) first before combining medications. LDL should be lower than 100, if possible, in order for cholesterol plaques to recede.

Women with extremely elevated triglycerides (above 400) sometimes respond quite well to gemfibrozil along with diet control and abstinence from alcohol (alcohol tends to increase the triglyceride level). High triglycerides is now found to be an important risk factor for women and men to develop coronary artery disease.

As in all medications, there can be dozens of side effects in about 1 to 3 percent of those taking them, including gastrointestinal complaints, depression, allergic reactions, and blood disorders.

Patients should be aware that all the studies of cholesterol-lowering medications had some bizarre findings. There was a higher-than-expected rate of death from suicide and accidental trauma among patients taking cholesterol-lowering drugs, although the heart-attack death rate decreased dramatically. As yet, there is no explanation for the suicides and traumas, which occurred primarily among male subjects, and this finding has to be confirmed.

European studies have alerted us to another strange finding. Patients whose cholesterol was below 160 had a higher incidence of cancer. Most researchers feel it is not the low cholesterol that caused the cancer, but that the cancer somehow affected the level of cholesterol in the blood. This is another area of research that is being conducted at this very moment.

VITAMIN E. As noted in Chapter 3, LDL cholesterol is recognized as one of the major culprits in coronary artery disease. Vitamin E appears to prevent LDL oxidation. In a study of 87,000 American female nurses conducted by the Nurses' Health Study in Boston, vitamin E lowered the heart-attack rate by 46 percent, apparently because of its antioxidant powers. The dosage given was 100 IU (international units) daily.

VITAMIN C. Women with the highest intake of vitamin C had lower rates of coronary artery disease than women with lower intakes, according to an eight-year study of 245 women at Brigham and Women's Hospital in Boston. The amount of vitamin C needed to reduce the heart-disease risk has not been established, however. Double Nobel laureate Linus Pauling, Ph.D., recommends 10 grams per day or more of vitamin C. But again, more study is needed.

BETA-CAROTENE. Diets high in beta-carotene, another antioxidant, were studied at Harvard University Medical School, using 12,900 subjects. People who received large amounts of beta-carotene had a markedly reduced death rate from cardiovascular disease, the study found.

Raw carrots, spinach, sweet potatoes, dried apricots, and cantaloupes are among the best sources of beta-carotene. Some doctors recommend one beta-carotene pill (25 IU) per day. Studies of beta-carotene are continuing.

I recommend that all women get plenty of vitamins C

and E, beta-carotene, and folic acid from their diet or from supplements as a preventive measure. I make the same recommendation to women with established coronary artery disease. Unfortunately, there are no official guidelines as to how much of these nutrients beyond the minimum daily requirement are needed to protect the heart.

DRUGS THAT REDUCE THE HEART ATTACK RISK

ASPIRIN. Aspirin has been used as a pain reliever for 2,500 years. In its pure form, aspirin, or acetylsalicylic acid (ASA), is not tolerated well by the stomach. In 1892, chemist Felix Hoffman refined pure aspirin so his father could take it to relieve his severe arthritis pain. Hoffman sold his refined drug to the Bayer Company in Germany, which labeled the new product aspirin. Today in the United States alone, over fifteen thousand tons of aspirin are taken annually.

Until recently, pain relief was the primary, if not the sole reason people took aspirin. In 1971, scientists discovered another property: Aspirin interferes with the blood's ability to clot. Numerous studies, which unfortunately included only men, have since suggested that a daily low dose of aspirin reduced the incidence of a first heart attack in those suffering from angina by 44 percent.

To be effective in reducing heart attacks, you need only a small dose of aspirin. Large dosages do not help and can be harmful. I recommend either a baby aspirin every day, or half of a 325 mg coated aspirin every day to women who smoke and who have low HDL, high LDL, diabetes, or angina.

Patients with prolonged angina at the beginning of a

heart attack are advised to take half an aspirin even as they are being transferred to the emergency room. Aspirin also is used in emergency rooms along with clot-busting drugs (see Chapter 4).

One of aspirin's most common and serious side effects is bleeding in the stomach. Also, there was higher-than-usual incidence of brain hemorrhages and strokes in all the aspirin studies to date.

Women are generally cautioned against taking aspirin during pregnancy and delivery because it can increase the risk of fetal hemorrhage and maternal bleeding. A pregnant woman should confer with her obstetrician to receive proper guidance on the use of aspirin during pregnancy.

In addition to its cardiovascular benefits, aspirin may possibly decrease the risk of colon cancer, a recent study suggested.

BETA-BLOCKERS. Cells in your heart, blood vessels, lungs, and muscles have receptors called "beta-adrenergic receptors." When stimulated, these receptors produce adrenaline-like chemicals. Adrenaline has both good and bad effects. It causes the heart to race, its contractions to increase, ups the flow of blood from the heart, and can save your life if you need a burst of energy or strength. Adrenaline is central to the flight or fight reflex that all mammals have. For example, if you must run to avoid an oncoming train, adrenaline helps propel you from danger by giving more force to your heart's contractions.

Drugs that block the action of the beta-adrenergic receptors are called beta-blockers. Beta-blockers cause blood pressure to fall, the pulse to slow, and allow the heart to function with less oxygen.

Beta-blockers have been used since 1971 for the treatment of angina and high blood pressure. Beta-blockers are given to some patients during or after a heart attack. Some studies have shown that beta-blockers, when taken after a heart attack, may reduce the chances of a second heart attack by 40 percent.

Another potential use for beta-blockers is to treat silent ischemia, a serious condition which was discussed in Chapter 8.

Beta-blockers also can offset the fast heartbeat, blood pressure rise, and surge of adrenaline that occur during bouts with anger. Women who are easily angered may need beta-blockers because this strong emotion causes the heart to race, the blood pressure to rise, and can precipitate angina and even a heart attack. Psychotherapy for stress reduction also is helpful in controlling anger. Anger is worth controlling because some studies have suggested doing so may help reverse coronary artery disease.

Some commonly prescribed beta-blockers include metoprolol, propranolol, timolol, atenolol, and nadolol.

As a group, beta-blockers are excellent medications, but there are potentially untoward effects. In my practice, women tolerate beta-blockers better than men do, although libido may be decreased and orgasm retarded in some women. In most men, beta-blockers cause impotence.

Women with asthma or severe lung disease are advised to avoid beta-blockers because they cause the bronchial passages to constrict. Women with peripheral vascular disease will find that their leg pain becomes worse when they take a beta-blocker.

Sometimes, beta-blockers will cause the pulse to become too slow and the blood pressure to fall. When this happens, the patient may experience a fainting spell. This is especially true in warm weather, when the blood vessels dilate and the fluid intake is often inadequate. In such cases, patients are usually admitted to the hospital and observed for about twenty-four hours to make certain that it was the medication—and not something else—that caused the fainting episode.

Many patients who take beta-blockers experience fatigue and conclude that their exhaustion originates from their heart being weakened. Older women often interpret drug-induced fatigue as a sign of aging. You should report any symptom to your physician, even if you don't think it's attributable to the drug you are taking.

Patients who engage in an exercise program may tire faster while taking beta-blockers, so they should adjust their exercise regimes accordingly. I play tennis with a middle-aged woman who takes a beta-blocker for angina. Her game starts slowly, but by the third or fourth game, she overcomes the drug's effect and becomes a tyrant on the court. Once blockers are discontinued, patients find that their energy level returns.

I cannot overemphasize the importance of never halting treatment with beta-blockers, or any cardiovascular medication, on your own. Cutting off beta-blockers abruptly can cause a dangerous rise in blood pressure or bring on a heart attack. Your physician must wean you off the drug by gradually reducing the dosage over several days or a week.

CALCIUM CHANNEL BLOCKERS. Calcium, a mineral, is needed for the contraction of smooth muscles of the heart and arteries. Calcium channel blocking agents prevent the calcium from entering the cells of the heart and blood vessels. As a result, the heart muscle relaxes and the blood vessels dilate, increasing the blood supply to the heart and decreasing its workload. This relieves angina. Calcium blockers also are used to treat peripheral vascular disease, hypertension, spasms of the coronary arteries, and Syndrome X (see Chapter 2).

Experiments have suggested that calcium channel blockers may impede the formation of cholesterol plaque and even help these artery-clogging plaques regress.

Women who take calcium supplements to prevent osteoporosis can take calcium carbonate, which does not adversely affect the cardiovascular system.

A combination of nitroglycerine patches, beta-blockers, and calcium channel blockers are commonly used to treat angina and are given after a heart attack. Some channel blockers, such as verapamil, also are used to regulate abnormal heart rhythms.

Channel blockers have side effects. For women, the most annoying one is ankle swelling. If you have varicose veins, nifedipine (Adalat, Procardia) can cause increased ankle swelling. Headaches and dizziness are other common side effects.

Verapamil and diltiazem both can cause slowing of the heart. If, in addition to these drugs, you are also using a beta-blocker, the combination can sometimes cause serious slowing of the heart, or even heart block and fainting. As soon as the medications are stopped, the heart rate returns to normal.

CHAPTER 12

ESTROGEN

In the 1940s, researchers gave menopausal women estrogen taken from pregnant mares. The women enjoyed dramatic relief from hot flashes. That finding launched what has become an almost billion-dollar estrogen-replacement industry. Fifteen to 20 percent of women suffer intense menopause symptoms, and up to 20 percent of them are taking estrogen replacement to relieve those symptoms.

A ten-year study of 49,900 nurses, part of the Nurses' Health Study in Boston, concluded in the late 1980s that estrogen has even more far-reaching benefits. Women who took estrogen after menopause cut their heart-attack risk by 50 percent.

Estrogen production by the ovaries begins its slow decline around age thirty-five. By age forty-five to fifty-five, estrogen production is almost gone and menopause begins. The ovaries still produce some estrogen after menopause, but probably not enough to provide cardiovascular protection.

The withdrawal of estrogen also adversely affects the vagina, vulva, uterus, breasts, skin, bones, and the heart. Stress incontinence can arise from the loss of lining of the bladder and the weakening of the pelvic muscles. Sexual intercourse can become painful due to a lack of lubrication, and there may be postcoital bleeding.

After menopause, the bones lose calcium and other minerals and begin to thin out. If bone density becomes low enough, there is the constant threat of fractures of the pelvis, hip, and other bones. Hip fractures in older women have a relatively high mortality rate because of the complications stemming from hip surgery.

As the estrogen level drops, so does the good cholesterol, HDL. At the same time, the level of LDL, the killer cholesterol, rises. Estrogen replacement helps preserve the healthier premenopausal HDL/LDL ratio.

Recent studies of the coronary arteries showed that postmenopausal women taking estrogen had a lower risk of severe blockage of the coronary arteries because their HDL levels were higher. Estrogen also increases blood flow because it dilates the arteries.

According to an analysis reported as part of the Nurses' Health Study in 1987, women treated with 0.625 or 1.25 mg of estrogen daily had a 50 percent reduction in coronary death as compared to nontreated women.

ESTROGEN RISKS. While there is little argument that estrogen reduces the risk of heart disease, there is evidence that estrogen replacement also increases the incidence of breast and uterine cancer somewhat. Studies are still in progress to determine the effects and safety of estrogen treatment. For now, I urge women to individualize their estrogen needs by consulting their doctors.

Most doctors will dissuade a woman from taking estrogen if she has a strong family history of breast cancer.

For example, a woman whose sister, mother, and aunt had breast cancer is at greater risk of developing cancer of the breast even without estrogen replacement. With estrogen, her risk may be even higher. Women who have had a mastectomy also are urged to shy away from estrogen, even if the cancerous breast was removed decades earlier.

ESTROGEN AND BLOOD PRESSURE. Studies have shown that estrogen replacement lowers blood pressure. Don't confuse estrogen replacement with birth control pills, which can raise the blood pressure.

PROGESTERONE. Progesterone is another female hormone produced by the ovaries. Oral progesterone often is added to estrogen-replacement therapy because progesterone lowers the risk of uterine cancer. Progesterone has a significant downside, however. This hormone reduces HDL and is believed to make the arteries more prone to arteriosclerosis. These problems may offset the good cardiovascular effects of estrogen.

If you have had a hysterectomy, progesterone is not needed and should not be taken. When progesterone is called for, it should be prescribed in the lowest possible dose.

CHAPTER 13

TREATING ANGINA

Angina, the wrenching chest pain usually caused by reduced blood supply to the heart muscle, afflicts an estimated 2 to 3 million women, primarily older, in the United States. This chapter will explore both medicinal and nonmedicinal treatments to stave off an angina attack and cope with one when it strikes.

PREVENTING AND RELIEVING ANGINA WITHOUT DRUGS

For many women, angina episodes are somewhat predictable. They may come after large meals, in cold weather, or during emotional upsets. By paying attention to the circumstances surrounding your angina attacks, you will get to know your body better and be able to prevent angina in many instances.

If you smoke and suffer angina, the suggestions that follow are less likely to help you. Smoking increases hardening of the arteries and causes spasms of all the arteries. In the heart, these spasms can cause angina.

If your angina attack comes after a large meal, try eating smaller and more frequent meals. The diet described in the last chapter of this book has helped many women suffering from angina, probably because it helped reverse blockages in their coronary arteries.

Covering your mouth with a scarf can prevent angina that is triggered by breathing cold winter air, which can cause spasms of the arteries.

The coronary arteries are very sensitive to our emotions. Laughter and joy relax them. Stress and anxiety cause them to go into spasms. An unpleasant confrontation, aggravation, frustration, rushing to beat a deadline, meeting your prospective in-laws ("in-law angina"), and numerous other stressful situations can cause angina. Anger, in particular, is an albatross for patients with angina, and has even caused heart attacks in some angina sufferers.

If your angina seems to come on the heels of emotional upheaval, consider some lifestyle changes. Give yourself extra time to get to the airport or to your office instead of rushing everywhere, for example. Having a cushion of time can prevent you from getting angry if you get caught in traffic.

If you can learn to laugh more each day, you may find that your angina episodes become less frequent. Rather than losing your temper or nagging your husband or kids, look for the absurdity in your response and laugh at yourself instead.

Another way of averting stress-induced angina is to simplify your life. One tactic might be getting rid of your telephone's call-waiting feature if you get stressed out juggling two conversations at once.

As much as possible, avoid anxiety-provoking situations or people. Ask yourself why a particular situation is causing you to become angry or anxious. Sometimes, the answer will help you cope better the next time.

In this regard, angina can have positive effects. Angina is a great excuse to reexamine your life and your relationships and to put your emotional house in order. Taking steps to avoid angina may actually improve your quality of life.

Make time to do the things you enjoy but always put off. One patient of mine always wanted to take up drawing, so she joined an art class. Another patient used to dream of seeing her words in print and got a local newspaper to publish one of her articles. Both women had angina and were under constant stress. Although they had to continue working their full-time jobs, they gained inner peace through their new activities. In both cases, the angina disappeared.

Another way to find inner peace is simply by rediscovering the wonders around you. Visit a museum you haven't been to in years, or spend time in your local library. What can be more relaxing than marveling at a painting or reading a classic?

Some women, after being diagnosed with angina, fear any form of exercise. They may even avoid sex because they are afraid to exert themselves and precipitate a heart attack. In the vast majority of cases, such fears are unwarranted. Indeed, being sexually satisfied is a means of achieving relaxation. Perhaps more essential is a graded exercise program. It need not be strenuous. Walking is a delightful form of exercise. Walking or other mild exercise will keep your weight down, assist in lowering your blood pressure, and strengthen your heart. Using the exercise stress test, your doctor can advise you on how much exercise you can do safely.

MEDICATIONS TO TREAT ANGINA

NITROGLYCERIN. Nitroglycerin is the oldest drug used to relieve angina. Nitroglycerin is also dynamite. It was discovered in 1876 by Alfred Nobel, for whom the Nobel Prize is named. Nitroglycerin's medicinal value was discovered in Nobel's explosives-manufacturing factory, where many employees got severe headaches, but workers with angina got relief from chest pain.

Around the same time, Thomas Bunton, a young surgeon in Edinburgh, poured some of the liquid explosive on a handkerchief and gave it to an angina patient to inhale. Chest pain was relieved almost immediately.

Nitroglycerin relieves angina because it widens the arteries and allows the heart to receive greater amounts of oxygenated blood. Nitroglycerin also dilates the veins throughout the body. This means that less blood returns to the heart, making the heart smaller and in need of less oxygen to contract. All these responses happen very quickly, relieving angina pain in minutes. Countless angina patients have enjoyed a better quality of life thanks to nitroglycerin.

The drug is administered as a fine tablet under the tongue, as a pill that is swallowed, or as a paste or patch placed on the chest. It also can be given intravenously in a hospital during a heart attack.

SIDE EFFECTS. Some patients suffer a furious headache from the first dosage of nitroglycerin. Headaches continue to be common when taking nitroglycerin in tablet form or by skin patch. The headaches usually subside after the medication is used for a couple of weeks. Aspirin, acetaminophen, or ibuprofen can be taken along with the nitroglycerin pill or patch in order to relieve the headache.

Nitroglycerin can make patients feel giddy and weak because it precipitates a drop in blood pressure. The first dosage of nitroglycerin is best given sitting, in the event that the patient is very sensitive to it and has a drop in blood pressure sharp enough to make him or her faint.

Nitroglycerin is occasionally used in anticipation of an angina attack, as before sexual activity, or before going for a walk after a full dinner.

How many doses of nitroglycerin are needed varies from patient to patient. If you use too many nitroglycerin tablets each day, your doctor may decide you might be better off with bypass surgery or a balloon dilation of the artery.

Angina pain that does not subside with nitroglycerin is a danger signal. If this happens, call your doctor or go to a hospital as soon as possible because a heart attack may be imminent or in progress. Some patients are instructed to place a second nitroglycerin pill under their tongue. If they still have no relief, they should go to the hospital. These patients are accustomed to their angina and know how many nitroglycerin tablets it usually takes to bring relief.

Nitroglycerin is a volatile chemical that deteriorates after several months, especially in a warm climate. The drug is packaged in a dark bottle and should be kept in a cool place to preserve its potency. I have seen patients carry the same old bottle for years in their pocketbooks, long after the drug has ceased being effective.

BETA-BLOCKERS. Beta-blockers (see Chapter 11) have been used since 1971 to treat angina and high blood pressure. When combined with nitroglycerin patches, beta-blockers are quite effective in controlling angina.

CALCIUM CHANNEL BLOCKERS. The calcium channel blocker, nifedipine, was used in Europe to treat angina for at least ten years before it was approved for use in the United States. This class of drugs may be used alone or in combination with other medications to control angina (see Chapter 11).

CHAPTER 14

BALLOON ANGIOPLASTY

Balloon angioplasty—technically known as percutaneous transluminal coronary angioplasty or PTCA—was perfected in 1976 by Dr. Andreas Gruntzig of Stockholm. PTCA's goal is to open clogged coronary arteries without resorting to open-heart surgery. In the first few years after its introduction, about three thousand balloon angioplasties were performed in the United States. By 1991, that number had soared to at least 300,000.

During the procedure, a long, flexible tube called a catheter is inserted into the artery in the upper thigh and snaked to the aorta. From the aorta, the catheter is threaded into the opening of a coronary artery that is narrowed or blocked by cholesterol plaque. A guide wire is then passed through the catheter and beyond the obstruction.

Once the guide wire is in place, a special angioplasty catheter, with a tiny balloon on its tip, is passed along the wire. When it reaches the blocked coronary artery, the balloon is inflated at various pressures, squashing the plaque against the artery's wall, much as you might flatten a tomato with your palm. In most cases, the balloon opens the artery and blood flows more freely through the now unobstructed channel.

Balloon angioplasty should not be confused with cardiac catheterization and angiography, one of the diagnostic tests described in Chapter 5. While they both utilize catheters that are placed into the heart, angiography and angioplasty are not generally performed at the same time, unless it is an emergency. The reason is that doctors need time to interpret the results of the angiography and discuss treatment options and risks with the patient before proceeding.

Balloon angioplasty takes longer than catheterization and angiography—two to four hours, depending on how many arteries need to be opened and how responsive they are to the treatment. Some blocked arteries are relatively easy to open. If one artery has too many blocked areas, or if it is very twisted or too small, it may be impossible to open with the balloon.

The best results are achieved when the patient's arteries are relatively straight and there is a single plaque blockage that is no larger than the balloon itself. If the plaque formation is recent, it will be softer and more likely to respond to flattening. Up to two blocked arteries can be submitted to balloon angioplasty at a given time.

It appears that angioplasty is generally more successful in men than in women. This is because women's arteries tend to be smaller and more twisted, although some men's arteries also are small and twisted. Balloon angioplasty tends to be less successful in diabetics because they usually have more extensive coronary artery disease, and in obese individuals because it's more difficult to put the catheters in place.

According to the National Heart, Lung and Blood

Registry, the initial success rate of angioplasty approaches 90 percent. By success, we mean the blockage is reduced to 30 percent or less, and the flow of blood through the vessel is markedly increased.

RISKS. While angioplasty undoubtedly has prolonged many lives, it is far from perfect. Some 30 to 50 percent of women who undergo balloon angioplasty suffer a reblock of the widened artery (restenosis) within six months. About 4 percent of patients experience a reblock of the artery within forty-eight hours after the balloon dilation.

To lower the risk of reblockages, the patient must make a series of follow-up visits to her cardiologist and adhere to a program of preventive care, which usually consists of a low-fat diet, exercise, medication, and for smokers, smoking cessation. Unfortunately, even in patients who take excellent care of themselves, blockages will sometimes recur. Doctors are experimenting with different medications, trying to find a solution to prevent the plaque from forming again.

In about 5 percent of cases, a coronary artery that was 90 percent blocked goes into spasm or hemorrhages and becomes 100 percent obstructed during the angioplasty attempt. When this happens, an emergency bypass operation may be necessary to prevent damage to the heart. Balloon angioplasty, therefore, is best performed at a medical center approved to perform coronary bypass operations. The death rate from balloon angioplasty is about 1 percent, as it is for bypass surgery.

One avoidable complication is bleeding at the catheter's point of entry into the artery of the thigh. To prevent bleeding, the patient must lie still with her leg straight for a good twelve hours after the catheter is removed.

As newer techniques develop, the success rate for angioplasty will undoubtedly increase. Lasers and other methods of getting rid of the plaque are being investigated to supplement or replace the balloon.

Even in its current state of evolution, angioplasty is considered a safe and cost-effective alternative to open-heart surgery for many patients. Successful balloon dilations make it possible for the patient to leave the hospital in a few days and return to a productive life, free from chest pain.

WHO IS A CANDIDATE FOR BALLOON ANGIOPLASTY?

Generally, balloon angioplasty is indicated when only one or two coronary arteries are severely blocked or narrowed. If all three coronary arteries are blocked, bypass surgery is the treatment of choice.

Balloon angioplasty candidates include patients with stubborn angina that does not improve with dietary changes and medications.

Balloon angioplasty also can be performed during a heart attack in cases where the patient continues to have chest pain in spite of receiving intravenous nitroglycerin, and her condition is deteriorating. Emergency angioplasty is carried out, but the risk of complications under these dire circumstances is substantially greater than if the procedure had been scheduled in advance.

After a heart attack, an exercise thallium stress test and, if warranted, a cardiac catheterization and angiography should be done before the patient leaves the hospital. If these tests reveal that one or two coronary arteries are partially blocked, there is a danger of another attack. The patient may then be given a choice: balloon angioplasty, bypass surgery, or a trial of medications, such as nitroglycerin, beta-blockers, channel blockers, and aspirin. A strict nonfat diet should accompany all of these options.

Sometimes after a heart attack, angina reappears. In these cases, cardiac catheterization is usually performed, and if the blocked arteries appear amenable to balloon dilation, angioplasty is considered. If angina returns after the first balloon angioplasty, the procedure can be repeated a second time and even a third time. If angina returns again, I would recommend bypass surgery.

As discussed earlier, stress tests in women patients are notoriously difficult to interpret if they are abnormal, and angiography remains the gold standard to decide whether balloon angioplasty is indicated. If there is evidence of blockage of the artery then balloon angioplasty is again considered.

Balloons also can be used to open clogged arteries in the leg in patients with peripheral vascular disease.

One recent study acknowledged that too many balloon angioplasties are being performed in this country. Anyone with reservations about the procedure should get a second opinion.

All things considered, balloon angioplasty is an important weapon in the medical arsenal for the treatment of blocked arteries. Under the right conditions, I recommend angioplasty, as long as the patient understands all the risks and benefits.

CASE STUDY IN BALLOON ANGIOPLASTY

For six months, Jennifer, fifty-seven, suffered chest pain suggestive of angina. She could not tolerate nitroglycerin but got some relief from a beta-blocker. The beta-blocker caused considerable fatigue, however.

I gave her an exercise thallium stress test, which turned

out to be abnormal. She actually developed chest pain during the test, and the changes on her electrocardiogram confirmed the problem.

I then ordered a cardiac catheterization and angiography, which disclosed that she had a 90 percent blockage in her left descending artery. This artery supplies most of the front of the heart, and if it becomes 100 percent blocked, a patient such as Jennifer would risk losing most of her heart muscle.

The following day, she underwent balloon angioplasty. Four days later, she was discharged from the hospital, free from chest pain. I repeated the thallium stress test one week later, and the results were normal. A week after that, she was back at work.

Now it was up to her to change her lifestyle. She stopped smoking, and her gynecologist placed her on estrogen and progesterone. She followed the diet described in Chapter 21 and started on a moderate exercise program. Each day, she took a baby aspirin, vitamins E and C, beta-carotene, and folic acid.

Three months after her balloon angioplasty, Jennifer's cholesterol had dropped to 250, her HDL had risen to 40, and her LDL had fallen to 180—all major improvements from her previous blood tests. Because her LDL was still high, I also prescribed the cholesterol-lowering drug Simastatin. Six months after her angioplasty, Jennifer's LDL had dropped to 110.

At the end of two years, Jennifer felt marvelous, and her last exercise stress test was completely normal.

PREVENTION

Not all angioplasty results are as gratifying as Jennifer's. As mentioned earlier, as many as 50 percent of women who undergo balloon angioplasty experience restenosis, even among those who say they followed a low-fat diet and took their medication diligently.

I believe the main problem is that too many patients don't do enough to prevent coronary artery disease before or after angioplasty. Sometimes it is the doctor's fault for failing to outline a solid prevention program. Too many angioplasty patients leave the hospital with no clear diet or exercise program to follow. Many patients think that now that their artery is opened, they are free and clear to do whatever they wish. Then there are the patients who follow a low-fat diet for the first few months, but then revert to the poor eating habits that helped cause their atherosclerosis in the first place.

I am optimistic that the angioplasty success rate would increase, in nondiabetics at least, if more patients would adhere to a strict preventive program, refrain from smoking, and take estrogen-replacement therapy if they can.

CHAPTER 15

CORONARY ARTERY BYPASS SURGERY

As its name implies, the purpose of coronary artery bypass surgery is to bypass obstructed arteries in order to restore adequate blood flow to the heart muscle.

At the beginning of the surgery, the patient is put on a heart-lung machine. An artery from the chest (the internal mammary artery) or a vein from the leg is removed and reconnected between the aorta and a point on the coronary artery downstream past the obstruction. If multiple grafts are needed, both the mammary artery and leg vein may be used.

Depending on the number of arteries to be bypassed, the operation can take anywhere from one and a half to three hours or longer. After discharge from the hospital, the patient usually enters a cardiac rehabilitation program, where she can regain her strength under medical supervision.

Each year in the United States more than 200,000 bypass operations are performed. The operation's death rate is reportedly under 1 percent in most medical centers that have a long track record for such operations. At least 90 percent of patients who undergo bypass surgery no longer suffer from angina.

WHO IS A CANDIDATE FOR BYPASS SURGERY?

The heart muscle gets its nourishment from three arteries—the coronary arteries. If all three are critically blocked and the patient is suffering from angina, bypass surgery is the treatment of choice.

Another time to perform bypass surgery is when the left main coronary artery is more than 75 percent blocked. The left main artery supplies most of the blood to the left side of the heart. In these cases, balloon angioplasty (see Chapter 14) is too dangerous because the balloon can close off the artery, which destroys the left side of the heart and kills the patient.

Bypass surgery is performed on an emergency basis if angioplasty has failed, or, in some cases, if the patient has a heart attack and goes into shock. The latter is a new approach to treating of shock induced by a massive heart attack.

When bypass surgery is scheduled, it is considered elective surgery.

GENDER BIAS. The disparities in heart care given to men and women become most stark when the possibility of bypass surgery enters the picture. For a variety of reasons discussed in Part I of this book, women are less likely than men to receive exercise stress tests and the other diagnostic evaluations that help a physician decide whether to recommend bypass surgery.

In my own practice, it is often like pulling teeth to get an able-bodied older woman to take an exercise stress test. "I am too old and too tired to bother with all this nonsense," is the most common excuse I hear from patients not wanting to be submitted to diagnostic cardiac studies. Consequently, the diagnosis of any heart disease is delayed, and treatment becomes more difficult. With education, I believe this attitude is beginning to change, with fewer women waiting until the eleventh hour to get tested for heart disease.

Another reason most bypass operations have been performed on men is because their heart disease tends to surface at a earlier age, before there is extensive damage to the heart. Women usually don't develop clinical evidence of coronary artery disease until much later, usually when they are over age sixty. By the time such women come to surgery, they are more likely to have other medical problems, such as long-standing hypertension, kidney failure, stroke, or diabetes. These problems make bypass surgery more risky.

There also are socioeconomic reasons why women have fewer bypass operations. Often, older women live alone because they are widowed or divorced. Many live solely on Social Security and may not have enough money left over for health care beyond the incomplete coverage provided by Medicare. Older women tend to become less physically active, they may eat more, and drink more alcohol, and many do not go to a doctor at all, even a gynecologist. In most cases, these women have no Significant Other to encourage them to take better care of their health. They tend to be worried about osteoporosis and breast cancer and don't realize that heart attack is the number one killer of women.

In the past, another factor dissuading women from undergoing bypass surgery was negative press coverage. It was reported that bypass surgery results were worse for women than for men. Today, I believe this view is no longer justified. Each year, thanks to a variety of medical advances, coronary bypass surgery becomes safer and the success rate improves. This is especially true for female patients, whose hearts are finally beginning to get the medical attention they deserve. In almost every instance, surgery not only prolongs life, it also provides a dramatic improvement in a person's quality of life.

RISKS. As with clot-busting drugs and angioplasty, the purpose of bypass surgery is to save the heart from being damaged or destroyed, and to cure angina. Unfortunately, in about 3 percent of cases, bypass surgery causes a heart attack during the operation, and as a result the heart gets damaged.

If the damage is severe enough, and the heart loses its ability to contract efficiently, chronic heart failure can result (see Chapter 16). A few patients suffer so much damage to their heart that they require a heart transplant to survive (see Chapter 17).

Keep in mind that any operation, ranging from a tooth extraction to bypass surgery, can have complications. Hemorrhages can occur, albeit not that often. Stroke has been reported in up to 2 percent of bypass surgery patients. In rare instances, the patient cannot be taken off the heart-lung machine because the heart does not restart after the arteries are bypassed. A heart transplant may then be necessary.

Cigarette smokers, who have damaged lung tissue and produce abnormal amounts of mucus, are prime candidates for pneumonia following surgery.

ALTERNATIVES TO BYPASS SURGERY

As discussed earlier, balloon angioplasty is an excellent alternative to bypass surgery in many cases (see Chapter

14). Angioplasty does not require open-heart surgery, and the recovery period is far shorter.

In certain cases where surgery or angioplasty is deemed to be too dangerous, or the patient decides against those procedures, medical treatment alone is the only alternative.

LIFE AFTER BYPASS SURGERY

I am always amazed by the speed with which most patients recover from bypass surgery. Several years ago, when bypass surgery was in its infancy, patients remained hospitalized for weeks. Today, most leave the hospital in ten days or so and are back at work within a few months. Inactive women who are overweight may take longer to recover. Patients with diabetes or lung disease also may take longer to recover because they are more prone to infections and their incisions may take longer to heal.

A successful bypass operation usually eliminates the need for heart medications. It also frees the patient from the constant fear of angina attacks. Thanks to the use of mammary artery grafts, 80 percent or more of bypass patients are free of coronary artery disease for ten years. Of course, these statistics are meaningful only if the patient does not smoke, gets adequate exercise, and follows the type of diet outlined in Chapter 21. Women past menopause should also be put on estrogen-replacement therapy, if possible.

DEPRESSION AFTER SURGERY. One of the common aftermaths of bypass surgery is depression. The reason for this is unclear. Of course, depression may have been present before the bypass operation was performed.

Depression interferes with good healing and the patient's ability to return to a better life. In my experience, depression after surgery is alleviated markedly with the help of antidepressants and a sympathetic doctor.

A problem is that depression after surgery often is not diagnosed. A depressed woman might complain only of fatigue, to which her doctor may respond: "It is common to be tired after any operation."

If, after surgery, you suffer from fatigue, sleep disturbance, loss of concentration, or memory loss, it may stem from depression. Try not to grow discouraged and wonder if the operation was worth all the agony. If you feel worse after surgery, it probably is due to residual aches and pains coupled with depression.

All patients going into bypass surgery should be informed that they may suffer from depression afterward. If you are aware that this can happen, you are more likely to recognize the symptoms and discuss them with your doctor.

OTHER POST-SURGERY SYMPTOMS. One of the more common post-bypass symptoms is pain in the legs, originating where the veins used in the operation had been removed. Time heals, and you can accelerate healing with a good exercise program. I instruct my patients to do a simple exercise each day, lifting from their heels to their toes, beginning with five heel-toe lifts and gradually working up to one hundred. Heel-toe lifts strengthen the calves and promote blood circulation in the legs.

Chest pain is another consequence of bypass surgery. During bypass surgery, the breast bone (sternum) is opened and then sutured closed. Everyone heals at a different pace. Pains in the chest from the sutured sternum can last a long time. A cardiologist will be able to tell if the chest pain is from the trauma of the surgery or whether—and this is only a slim possibility—it is a coronary artery becoming clogged again.

In the first six weeks or so, patients are cautioned against driving because a traffic accident can injure their chest wall before it is properly healed. At the end of the second month, I usually perform a stress test on the patient to measure the success of the surgery.

FOLLOW-UP CARE. I strongly recommend that women who undergo bypass surgery include their family doctor in their follow-up care. Follow-up care can be a critical factor in recovery. Don't leave yourself entirely in the hands of your surgeon or cardiologist. Often, the surgeon sees you briefly before the operation and possibly a couple more times afterward. Cardiologists are tuned in to your heart and cardiovascular system and may miss another health problem that would be caught by an internist or family physician who knows you well.

After surgery, it is essential that you enter into a cardiac rehabilitation program, which most hospitals offer. Rehabilitation specialists will be able to answer all your questions, help dispel any fears, and introduce you to a good exercise program.

Your cholesterol level should be measured about two months after surgery to get a better picture of your lipid profile. Soon after surgery, most patients have low cholesterol, which begins to rise a few months later.

Ninety percent of my bypass patients report feeling much better since their operation. They are back at work, play tennis or golf, some ski, others even go scuba diving. A few fly their own airplanes. It is important to realize, however, that neither bypass surgery nor angioplasty can halt the relentless progression of atherosclerosis. In order to stop progression and induce regression of cholesterol plaques, you must exercise, control your fat intake, and take cholesterol-lowering medications, if necessary.

COMMON QUESTIONS ASKED ABOUT BYPASS SURGERY

Will I miss the veins taken from my leg?

Removing the veins will not affect the state of your legs, except for some periodic aching and swelling.

Will I no longer have to take any medications?

There will be no need to take medications for angina, but one baby aspirin a day is advised to retard the return of blockages in the arteries. If the Kra Diet (Chapter 21) does not bring the LDL level cholesterol down, then I recommend cholesterol-lowering drugs.

Will surgery eliminate my palpitations?

If they are caused by blocked arteries, the palpitations may disappear. Otherwise, palpitations, as a rule, are not corrected by bypass surgery.

If my new coronary arteries become blocked, will I have to be operated on again?

It may be possible to open the blocked grafts with an angioplasty, but a repeat bypass operation is sometimes necessary. Most surgeons agree that 60 percent of the grafts may close by the tenth year after the initial surgery.

Will I be able to jog, swim, and play tennis as I did before the operation?

Most patients return to their previous level of physical activity.

Can I become pregnant and go through a delivery after surgery?

Pregnancy and delivery will probably be safer than ever for you.

When can I resume my sex life?

As a general rule, after you can climb one to two flights of stairs without pain, you can resume your sex life without too much difficulty (see Chapter 19).

CHAPTER 16

CONGESTIVE HEART FAILURE

The heart is a remarkable muscle. About the size of your fist, its unimpressive appearance belies the fact it is a perfectly designed instrument. Like all living organs and tissues, the heart muscle must receive oxygen, sugar, electrolytes, minerals, proteins, vitamins, and other nutrients through the blood. Without oxygen and nutrients, the heart will die.

Properly nourished, the heart muscle contracts strongly, propelling blood from its chambers to all parts of the body. It then relaxes and dilates, allowing blood to flow in from the lungs and other parts of the body. The average heart contracts and relaxes more than 2.5 billion times during an average person's lifetime.

If the heart muscle is damaged, its pumping action becomes less efficient. Damage can be caused by such things as long-term high blood pressure, infections, abnormal heart valves, thyroid ailments, alcohol abuse, heart attack, and, of course, atherosclerosis.

The weakened muscle, having lost much of its ability

to contract or relax, causes blood to back up into vessels of the lungs. The fluid from the blood then leeches into the lung tissue itself. This is called congestive heart failure (CHF) because the lungs and other organs become congested, like a sponge soaked with water. If the congestion happens suddenly, and the lungs become filled with fluid, it is called pulmonary edema.

CHF should not be confused with a heart attack (cardiac arrest), although a heart attack can cause heart failure. Cardiac arrest means the heart no longer pumps blood; heart failure means the heart still pumps blood but does it ineffectively.

As stated in previous chapters, the main purpose of thrombolysis, angioplasty, and bypass surgery is to save the heart muscle. Likewise, one of the main reasons to keep the blood pressure normal, besides avoiding strokes, is to prevent damage to the heart.

At least 2 million people in the United States have congestive heart failure, and more than half are women. Each year, at least eight out of one thousand Americans are diagnosed with CHF. CHF is on the rise, primarily because more hearts than ever are being saved. While advances in surgery and medication are prolonging life, some individuals are left with damaged hearts. This is true particularly in older women and men.

SYMPTOMS OF EARLY HEART FAILURE

The symptoms of early heart failure can be elusive and tricky to diagnose.

Fatigue, so common in our busy society, can be the first hint that congestive heart failure is developing. Molly is a case in point.

Molly had high blood pressure for twenty years and

was very overweight. In May 1993, she noticed that she tired quickly after gardening. She adjusted by sitting rather than kneeling, but she continued to feel drained of energy after a short time in her garden.

After many weeks of urging by her three daughters, Molly finally consulted her family physician. With an old stethoscope, her doctor heard the telltale sounds of heart failure in her lungs, which sounded like water running through a brook. He did not have to resort to any other tests to diagnose CHF. The cause was an enlarged heart due to long-standing high blood pressure.

With the treatments described later in this chapter, Molly's fatigue vanished, and she was back planting and weeding her garden. (Ironically, her garden contained a beautiful purple flower—foxglove [*Digitalis purpurea*]—which, for many hundreds of years, has been used to treat congestive heart failure.)

Aside from fatigue, another early warning sign of CHF is shortness of breath, the most common symptom of heart failure. At first, shortness of breath is noticeable during physical effort, such as climbing stairs. As heart failure progresses, shortness of breath occurs even at rest. Chronic lung ailments from smoking also can produce shortness of breath. A stethoscope, chest X ray, and a radionuclear scan of the heart (MUGA, see Chapter 5) can help distinguish between the two conditions.

Shortness of breath was the first sign that another patient of mine, Shirley, was suffering from CHF. Her odyssey began one evening when she was stricken with a heart attack. Shirley, sixty-seven, could not receive thrombolysis (clot-dissolving medication) because she didn't arrive at the hospital until the following morning. Her attack, caused by blockages in all three coronary arteries, was massive. Even after bypass surgery, Shirley's heart was still damaged.

A MUGA scan taken after the operation showed her heart was just limping along, contracting poorly. As a result, Shirley was short of breath while climbing stairs or even walking, and she suffered from severe fatigue.

For both Shirley and Molly, I prescribed the following treatment regimen, which is considered standard for patients with severe CHF:

- A strict low-salt, low-fat diet;
- A diuretic called Lasix to reduce the amount of fluid in the body;
- Digoxin (a form of digitalis) to make the heart contract more effectively; and
- A nitroglycerin patch to help decrease the amount of blood returning to the heart, relieving congestion.

The regimen also includes a new class of medications called angiotensin converting enzyme (ACE) inhibitors. When used in conjunction with the other medications, ACE inhibitors relieve shortness of breath, increase the patient's ability to exercise, and above all, prolong life dramatically. Before the advent of ACE inhibitors, half of all patients with heart failure died within five years. Today, this new medical therapy has significantly improved patients' quality of life and reduced the five-year death rate by 50 percent.

If CHF is caused by a diseased heart valve, replacement of the valve may be necessary to improve heart function. When the cause is blocked coronary arteries, balloon angioplasty or bypass surgery can very often ameliorate CHF.

With modern treatment of congestive heart failure, patients not only live longer, but much more comfortably.

CHAPTER 17

HEART TRANSPLANTS

The first human heart transplant was performed on a man on December 2, 1967, in Capetown, South Africa, by Dr. Christiaan Barnard. The donor heart came from a young woman. The first American heart transplant was performed at the Stanford Medical School in California on January 6, 1968, by Dr. Norman Shumway. The donor heart that went into Michael Kasperak also came from a woman, who died at age forty-three. In 1993, more than 2,085 heart transplantations were performed in the United States. In recent years, women have become just as likely as men to receive a donor heart.

A heart transplant is a last-ditch effort to save a person's life in cases where congestive heart failure has progressed to the point of end-stage heart disease, when neither bypass surgery nor medications can help. The severity of congestive heart failure is determined in part by a nuclear scan of the heart (the MUGA). In a normal MUGA scan, the ejection fraction is above 55 percent (see Chapter 5). End-stage heart disease will have an ejection fraction of

10 percent or less. Other tests, including cardiac catheterization, pulmonary function, kidney function, and psychiatric evaluations, also are used to help select potential donor-heart recipients.

The age limit for secondhand hearts used to be fifty-five. Today, people well beyond age sixty are getting heart transplants. Candidates must be free of cancer, severe lung disease, and not require insulin if they have diabetes. Other exclusions depend on the transplant center.

Primarily due to a lack of available donor hearts, only 50 percent of patients waiting for a new heart receive one. In most cases, the patient dies of heart failure while on the waiting list. The longer a patient has to wait for a heart, the poorer the operation's outcome because the patient's health often deteriorates during the waiting period. The amount of time spent on a waiting list for a heart transplant typically ranges from three weeks to three months. If the patient is on life support or in intensive care, it's not unusual to rack up a medical bill of $130,000 during the waiting period alone. Cost of the transplant operation can run $100,000 or more.

There are a myriad of ethical questions surrounding organ transplantation. One of the more difficult dilemmas is: Should the person who waited the longest get the next available heart even if he or she is the worst candidate for survival? This and other ethical questions are generally worked out on a case-by-case basis by the medical team.

Currently in the United States, about fifteen thousand people are waiting for heart transplants, even though there are potentially more than enough donors. Some fifty thousand people die each year on U.S. highways, and there is one homicide in this country every minute. The ideal donor is thirty-five or younger and has suffered brain death; there must be no heart disease or crushing chest injury. Because human donor hearts are so scarce, surgeons are experimenting with baboon hearts, which are, in many ways, comparable to human hearts.

The body's rejection of donor hearts, once a major problem, is now controlled in virtually all cases thanks to new antirejection drugs such as cyclosporine. There are potential, dangerous side effects to cyclosporine, however, such as high blood pressure, kidney and liver problems, and difficulty fighting off infections. These side effects are minimal, however, compared to the drug's benefits. Antirejection medications are expensive, however, and must be taken for the rest of the patient's life.

On November 21, 1992, the *New Haven Register* reported a successful heart transplant on a thirty-six-year-old woman at the Yale New Haven Hospital. This young woman was a smoker, had severely clogged arteries, and had already undergone bypass surgery. The woman could not be removed from the heart-lung machine because her heart was so damaged. She was placed on a mechanical device to keep her heart pumping while she awaited a donor. Twelve weeks later, she underwent a successful heart transplant and now is back home, enjoying every moment of her fully restored life.

An estimated 80 percent of heart recipients are still alive five years after their operation. Quite a few patients are still alive twenty years after receiving new hearts.

As exemplified by this woman, patients with a second-hand heart can lead active, productive lives. Many even return to vigorous physical activities, such as tennis, skiing, and swimming. (On the other hand, it's hard to believe, but more than 40 percent of heart recipients return to smoking, and the major cause of death in most of these cases is coronary artery disease.)

Until we can prevent coronary heart disease and other forms of heart muscle destruction, heart transplants will be here to stay.

CHAPTER 18

EXERCISE PRESCRIPTION FOR WOMEN

There is no doubt about it: When you engage in exercise on a routine basis, you feel better. People who exercise lose weight, strengthen their muscles, gain more flexibility, and are less prone to depression. Exercisers are more energetic during the day and tend to sleep better at night than do sedentary folk. Exercise raises the HDL (the guardian of our coronary arteries), lowers the LDL (the culprit of coronary artery disease), lessens premenstrual syndrome, curbs the urge to smoke, and adds to one's general sense of well-being.

Physical activity also strengthens the heart so it need not work as hard to circulate the blood. In time, regular exercise eventually decreases the resting and exercising pulse rates and lowers the blood pressure. The list of exercise benefits goes on and on. But suffice it to say that people who exercise regularly are apt to live longer, healthier, and more productive lives and have a greater chance of avoiding heart attacks than do couch potatoes.

Numerous research studies and observations, dating

from the ancient Greeks and Egyptians, testify to the benefits of exercise. Consider this statement made by a Greek doctor two thousand years ago: "Exercise ferments the humors [vital bodily fluids], casts them into their proper channels, throws off redundancies, gives vigor to the person, and allows the soul to act with cheerfulness."

WHAT KIND OF EXERCISE IS BEST?

According to Dr. William B. Kannel, head of the landmark Framingham Heart Study, exercise should:

- Give the woman pleasure and enjoyment. If, for example, you find jogging to be tedious or boring, try another form of exercise such as bicycling, tennis, or low-impact aerobics.
- Last about twenty minutes per session and be continuous.
- Be performed at least three times a week, or better yet, four or five times a week.

One of the most difficult problems doctors face is persuading female patients to exercise. Numerous studies have shown that up to 90 percent of women do no exercise at all. Of women who do begin an exercise program, 90 percent quit after a short period. Exercise must be sustained over many months in order to reap its beneficial effects.

Scores of sedentary women ages eighteen through fifty-five have told me they simply don't have enough time for exercise. This is especially true for career women with families. In many cases, their days begin as early as 6 A.M. and don't end until midnight. If you are in this category, my advice is to block out a mere three or four hours a week—a tiny percentage of the 168 hours in a week—for exercise and jealously guard that time. Try to schedule the same hours every week, and make no other commitments. If possible, invite your spouse, children, or a friend to join you. If someone else is involved in your exercise period, you are more apt to get on that bicycle or show up for that exercise class.

Some people, especially overweight women, hate exercise classes not because of the sweat, but because of vanity. Most aerobics classes are held in rooms with lots of mirrors and toned bodies, which makes some women self-conscious. Many overweight women make the mistake of comparing their body with others' and conclude they would rather stay fat than be seen in revealing exercise garb.

One solution is wearing loose shorts and a T-shirt instead of a bodysuit to class. Fight the tendency to compare yourself to others in a self-deprecating way. Instead, make a physically fit classmate your inspiration. Perhaps she started out flabby, too. Another alternative is to join or launch an exercise class just for overweight individuals. Find out if the hospital in your community sponsors a beginners' exercise class geared for the overweight, sedentary person. To start your own class (even if it's just a class of one), all you need is some space, a TV, VCR, and one of the dozens of quality exercise videos that are sold everywhere.

WHO SHOULD NOT EXERCISE

Not every woman should exercise. There are certain medical conditions that make exercise a potentially dangerous activity. Women who have a narrowing of the aortic valve (aortic stenosis) should not exercise because it can lead to sudden death. Women who suffer from angina or have sustained a recent heart attack are advised never to start an exercise program without consulting a doctor and undergoing an exercise stress test to determine what level their pulse rate can reach safely.

Smokers also are urged to check with their doctors and have a stress test. Smoking causes the arteries to go into spasms, which can trigger a heart attack during strenuous exercise.

Likewise, women with high blood pressure should have a stress test before embarking on an exercise program. The blood pressure may be well controlled under sedate conditions, but can leap to dangerous levels during exercise.

Agnes, a patient of mine with high blood pressure, had a stress test before taking up jogging—and it may have saved her life. During her test, her pulse increased to 110, and her blood pressure rose to 230 systolic and 130 diastolic—stroke levels. By adjusting her medications over a period of three months, she reached the point where she was able to safely engage in a prescribed (and limited) exercise program.

Anytime you are having chest pain, stop exercising and call your doctor immediately. One patient, while experiencing chest pain, decided to jog to see if the pain would become worse. It did. She had a massive heart attack that almost killed her.

I am against *strenuous* exercise for patients with heart disease or hypertension. Jogging five miles around a hilly neighborhood is strenuous exercise; jogging in place on a soft rug is not. In 1985, I wrote an article for the *New York Times* titled "Joggomania: The Secret of Longevity Does Not Lie in a Pair of Jogging Sneakers." I still hold this opinion. The majority of people who drop dead while jogging had coronary artery disease. Also, jogging will not prolong your life if you smoke and eat fatty foods, especially if your cholesterol level is elevated. Under these circumstances, jogging or any strenuous exercise program can be more hurtful than helpful.

EXERCISING SAFETY

After being cleared by your physician, here are some general guidelines to help you exercise safely:

- If you become dizzy or weak, stop exercising. Check with your doctor.
- Don't exercise directly after a meal. After eating, blood moves to your intestine to help digestion. If your heart, arm, and leg muscles begin demanding more blood at the same time, you can have a fainting episode, or worse.
- Avoid exercising in the heat of the day. When it is hot, the heart must work very hard. This can be dangerous for anyone suffering from angina or heart disease.
- Avoid exercising when you have a cold, have not slept well the night before, or drank too much alcohol the day before. Illness, alcohol, and fatigue depress your resistance to infections and could lead to fluctuations in blood pressure during exercise.

GETTING STARTED

If you have never exercised before, or haven't for a very long time, consider walking. Walking is a wonderful form of exercise for anyone, especially beginners. Walking two miles per hour (a fast walk) burns about 240 to 280 calories. Running two miles uses the same number of calories, but in a shorter period of time, and offers the same cardiovascular benefits.

I instruct my more ambitious patients who walk each day to wear a knapsack containing several books. Gradually increasing the book load improves posture and gives the heart an even better workout.

The American Heart Association walking program begins with one quarter-mile in eleven minutes the first week, one quarter-mile in eight minutes the second week, one half-mile in fifteen minutes the third week, and one mile in thirty minutes the fourth week. By the sixth week, those following this regimen should be able to walk one mile in twenty minutes. One mile is about twenty city blocks.

Walking two or three miles a day can do wonders. Some large indoor shopping malls open their doors to "mall walkers" before store hours so you can get your walking in during inclement weather. Mall walking any time of day is ideal for people who don't feel safe walking near their homes or can only find time to walk after sundown.

For safety reasons, it is usually a good idea to walk with a partner. A walking partner also can provide encouragement and companionship, making the time seem to pass faster.

If you have angina or have had a recent heart attack, try to walk on a level surface. Again, an exercise stress test can tell how much exercise you can do safely, and by what increments you can safely increase your activity.

If you are thinking about investing in home exercise equipment, consider a stationary bicycle. You can keep boredom at bay by placing your exercise bike in front of a television set or stereo. Listening to music can help you keep a steady pace. Some stationary bicycles have a built-in stand for a book or a magazine.

Approximate Calories Expended per Minute of Physical Activity

Badminton	7
Basketball	5
Bicycling: 6 mph	4
10 mph	7
12 mph	9
Bowling	4
Canoeing	4
Dancing: Aerobic	9
Ballroom	6
Square dancing	6
Dusting	3
Furniture polishing	6
Gardening	4
Golf, with Cart: Power	3
Pulling	5
Horseback riding (trotting)	6
Ice skating	7
Ironing	2
Jogging: 5 mph	8
7 mph	12
Jumping rope: Slow	7
Medium	9
Fast	11
Mopping floors	4
Roller skating	6
Rowboating	5
Rowing machine	5
Running: 8 mph	7
10 mph	13
Scrubbing floors	6
Skiing: Cross-country	11
Downhill, 10 mph	10

Squash and handball	10
Swimming	8
Table tennis	6
Tennis: Singles	7
Doubles	6
Vacuuming	4
Walking: 2 mph	3
3 mph	5
4 mph	7

Bicycling at six miles per hour burns four calories per minute. If you double your speed to twelve miles per hour, you will use up nine calories per minute.

Dancing is hardly boring and burns six calories per minute (unless you are doing a slow foxtrot—fun, but not exercise). Ballroom dancing also is great aerobic exercise.

If you're not a dancer, try jogging in place or jumping rope (on a padded carpet or no-skid rug) for ten minutes every morning. Each of these activities burns seven calories per minute. An easy way to meet your exercise goal is by jogging or dancing for ten to twenty minutes each morning four times a week. If you jump fast for ten minutes, you will burn eleven calories per minute. These short but frequent exercise sessions have a greater chance of becoming habitual because they can be done at home.

Chores are another type of physical activity that, by definition, are home-based. It's easy to forget how much energy it takes to keep a house tidy. Polishing furniture, for instance, uses six calories per minute; scrubbing floors burns six calories per minute; and dusting burns three calories per minute.

In general, exercise provides women with another important means of taking charge of their lives. This is especially true for heart-attack survivors and those who have undergone bypass surgery. For them, exercising regularly can instill confidence that their hearts are stronger than they thought. This helps alleviate fear of dying suddenly. Exercise can prove to these patients that by taking good care of their bodies, there's every reason to believe they'll be around for quite a while.

CHAPTER 19

SEX AND HEART DISEASE

Unfortunately, sex often becomes a frightening proposition for women who have undergone heart surgery, or have suffered a heart attack or angina. But sexual activity after recovery from surgery, a heart attack, or angina not only can be safe and enjoyable, it can actually improve the heart's function.

Sex is a terrific form of exercise. Depending on how you and your partner go about it, up to ten calories per minute or more are burned during sexual intercourse. Lovemaking increases the heart rate and blood pressure, providing a cardiovascular workout.

FIGHTING THE FEAR. Studies have confirmed that there is a decrease in sexual activity after angioplasty, bypass surgery, and heart attack because of fear that sex will precipitate a heart attack. This fear can inhibit the libido. Also suppressing the desire for sex may be pain from the surgical scars on the chest and legs after bypass surgery. For some women, their sex drive is overpowered by an aversion to letting their partners see their surgical scars.

In subtle or overt ways, your partner may be conveying his fear of harming you with sexual activity. One husband confided in me that he was actually afraid of ripping his wife's chest open. He is a big man and she a tiny woman. I assured him that the scenario he fears has never been reported. And I suggested that there are other positions besides the missionary position (him on top of her) that are also very safe and may be more comfortable. Needless to say, he was delighted to hear this.

If your doctor says you're able to have sex, but your partner is still afraid of hurting you, reassure him. Oral sex and masturbation also are safe following a successful angioplasty or bypass operation. As with intercourse, though, it's best to proceed slowly at first to instill confidence that nothing bad will happen.

HOW LONG SHOULD YOU WAIT? This is not to say it's okay to seduce your husband the moment you get home from the hospital after a heart attack. Here is a rule of thumb I tell my patients: If you can climb a flight of stairs without having chest pain or your pulse rate rising over 130, you can safely engage in sexual activities, with your doctor's approval.

Even if it's too soon to resume sexual activities, there's nothing wrong with hugging and caressing, so long as the hugs are gentle (a bear hug can hurt).

QUESTIONS ABOUT SEX MOST OFTEN ASKED BY HEART PATIENTS

Can an orgasm hurt my heart?

Orgasms will not harm your cardiac status. Nor have multiple orgasms been shown to be harmful. If you experience angina pains during sexual activity, however, your doctor should know about it. Your doctor may recommend another exercise stress test. Or you may be asked to wear a Holter monitor. If worn during orgasm, the monitor's ECG log will document whether angina was present. If the ECG tracing is abnormal, further diagnostic tests may be needed to determine whether angioplasty, bypass surgery, or a medication adjustment is necessary.

Can sexual activity harm my chest incision?

By the third week after surgery, the sutured chest is usually properly healed and cannot be harmed during sexual intercourse.

Why have I lost my desire for sex?

Depression and anxiety are probably the major reasons for decreased sexual desire after a heart attack or bypass surgery. In addition, medications such as beta-blockers often decrease sexual desire in women (as well as in men), and can sometimes cause depression.

As discussed previously, depression often goes unrecognized, masquerading as fatigue, loss of interest, or sleep disturbance. Sleep disturbance is one of the main keys used to diagnose depression. A depressed patient may have no trouble going to sleep, but she falls in and out of sleep throughout the night. In the morning, she feels exhausted, as if she hadn't slept at all. For the rest of the day, she feels tired and listless and may fear this means her heart is not functioning properly. If this is happening to you, an honest discussion with your doctor is essential.

Fortunately, depression after bypass surgery or a heart attack can be ameliorated dramatically with antidepressant medications. An antidepressant given at bedtime, for example, often lifts the depression within several weeks, allowing the libido to return.

Many people, after a heart attack or bypass surgery,

find their sexual desire is actually more intense than before their hospitalization. Mostly, these are the patients who are following a prudent dietary program, exercising regularly, and have quit smoking. Their libido increases because they no longer fear that they will die from a heart attack.

One delightfully vigorous woman asked me after bypass surgery when she could return to her sex life. I told her that if she could climb one or two flights of stairs without pain, she could start. She returned the following week and said her husband did not believe her. At her request, I wrote her a prescription stating: "Dear Mr. Jones, Your wife can engage in moderate sexual activity." She returned the following week and said, "He still won't believe me. Would you please write another prescription, but this time address it: 'To Whom It May Concern.' "

CHAPTER 20

HOW TO QUIT SMOKING

Smoking is the major cause of early death from heart disease, lung cancer, and cancer of the bladder. Regardless of what other steps you take to improve your health, heart disease cannot be stopped or reversed if you continue to smoke.

Hypnosis, copper bracelets, meditation, private pacts with God, psychotherapy, nicotine patches, nicotine gum, and smoking-cessation classes all are helpful—if you have made up your mind to quit. Studies have shown that a personal resolve to quit is the single most important factor, perhaps the only crucial factor, that determines whether you will succeed.

For some smokers, quitting cold turkey produces restlessness, anxiety, bad temper, drowsiness, sleep disturbance, and an inability to concentrate. These withdrawal symptoms are usually most intense during the first week and begin to subside after about three weeks. The reason most people relapse is because their craving for nicotine continues.

For the past twenty years, I have prescribed the following smoking-cessation technique to my patients. Most found it to be amazingly successful. If you truly want to give up smoking, read on. If not, I urge you to reread the chapter on heart attacks.

FOUR-WEEK PROGRAM TO QUIT SMOKING

As addictive as cigarettes are, it's important to realize that smoking is a learned habit, something that was practiced and reinforced until it became a reflex. Pick up the phone and you automatically reach for a cigarette; hold a cocktail, and reach for the cigarette; drink a cup of coffee, and you light up; a moment grows tense, reach for a smoke.

Most smokers learned to smoke from other smokers—probably parents and friends—as well as from advertisements, television shows, and movies. The Madison Avenue image of an elegant woman with her wide-brimmed hat and long white gloves, sitting seductively in a European café with her handsome lover, blowing clouds of smoke into his adoring face, makes smoking seem irresistibly sexy. But there is nothing romantic about poisoning your body with the dozens of toxic chemicals that make up tobacco smoke.

If you want to quit, you must work hard to break the vile habit. (It's as simple, and as hard, as that.) If your Significant Other also smokes, it will help if he or she participates in my program, too.

Before you get started, buy the following items: a gallon of good mouthwash, some string, wrapping paper, a pair of sneakers, and rock 'n' roll tapes or CDs (or any lively dance music).

Week One

Begin each morning with a spirited five-minute aerobic dance to music. Dancing in private affords you the luxury of being dressed or undressed, and can eliminate any feelings of self-consciousness. Singing while dancing further enhances the lung and heart workout.

At first, you may get short of breath. Don't be discouraged. In due time, your morning dance will become easier. If dancing makes you feel uncomfortable or embarrassed, jog in place or do any type of jumping exercise. If you have arthritis in your knees or ankles, try simulating a swim in the lake with the upper portion of your arms for five to ten minutes.

You can continue to smoke all you want, but you may not light up your first cigarette of the day until noon. This will help you break that morning smoking habit. Once you can tolerate not smoking before noon, you're on your way to quitting forever.

Use your mouthwash after breakfast and after every cigarette, or at least once an hour, even while you are at work. It is important that your mouth be free of smoke odor. Each evening, take a long shower to cleanse the traces of smoke and tobacco from your hair and body. (When I examine someone in my office, I can smell the stench of cigarettes or cigars, even as the patient is denying that he or she smokes.) Help clear the tobacco odor from your home by emptying and washing all your ashtrays every morning, and tuck them out of sight.

Week Two

This week, increase your morning aerobic exercise session to ten minutes. Scrub your body and nails to clean off smoke residue and tobacco stains. Smoke all you wish, but again, refrain from lighting up that first cigarette until noon.

At work, keep your cigarettes off your desktop (it helps if smoking is prohibited in your workplace).

At home, don't leave your cigarettes in the bedroom, sitting room, study, or kitchen. Keep your cigarettes in a broom closet, on the floor, or another inconvenient spot. If you live in a house, stow your cigarettes in the basement and put the matches or lighter on the highest shelf in your kitchen.

Each time you feel the urge to smoke, use your mouthwash first. Only then allow yourself to retrieve a single cigarette. While smoking, do not sit down. And make sure you are not in your kitchen, bedroom, living room, or any other place where you normally have a cigarette. Smoke in the basement, garage, or in the hallway, where it's not very comfortable.

If you own a car, you may carry cigarettes and matches, but you must keep them in the trunk. Remove the cigarette lighter and restrict yourself to matches. Toward the end of Week Two, remove all cigarettes from your house and put them in the trunk of your car. You may go out to your car to get a cigarette as often as you wish, but you may only use the matches in your kitchen.

Week Three

Follow the same routine as Week Two, smoking as often as you wish, following the restrictions. This week, however, put your cigarettes in wrapping paper and tie them with string. The giftlike package is kept in the previously designated areas. If it's after noon and you want a cigarette, you must go out to the car (or basement or broom closet), unwrap the package, remove one cigarette, rewrap the package and tie it up, then walk to the kitchen to get matches. If any friends or family members are in your home, you must smoke outside. Don't forget to rinse with mouthwash afterward.

Jumping through all these hoops in order to smoke may seem silly. But it forces you to think twice and to "work" to smoke instead of automatically grabbing a cigarette.

Week Four

By now, the reflex to smoke should be beginning to weaken. Stick to the routine established in Weeks Two and Three. But now, if you normally attend a cocktail hour, do something physical instead such as dance, walk, or have sex. Alcohol encourages smoking; so do coffee and other caffeinated drinks. Drink only decaffeinated coffee or tea.

During Week Four, skip the cigarettes you normally have after a meal or with your coffee. And remember to use mouthwash frequently. With your daily dancing routine (and all the exercise you're getting just to retrieve each cigarette), the level of nicotine in your system should be decreasing. The number of cigarettes you are smoking each day should be going down as well.

If you follow my program, you should be completely free of nicotine dependence by the end of Week Four. Your desire to smoke is likely to remain, but it should seem like too much trouble to go through all the acrobatics in order to do so. You will feel ridiculous having to unwrap a package of cigarettes only to rewrap it again. By this point, you should be able to recognize that cigarettes were your master and that you don't need them to relax, even after sex.

For the next two months, continue to use the mouthwash frequently and maintain your daily exercise program. The mouthwash helps rid you of the phantom residual smoke sensation in your mouth. You probably won't feel like smoking if you have a clean mouth and your exercise tolerance has increased. Exercising daily will prevent you from gaining weight and help curb your appetite. If you're like most of my patients who successfully quit smoking, you'll want to take up more strenuous exercises once you begin to slim down and breathe better. Healthy eating can further hasten your detoxification from nicotine. The diet described in Chapter 21 is designed to limit your caloric intake while decreasing your craving for cigarettes.

It doesn't take long after quitting for your energy level to increase. All the reserved energy that had been blunted by your smoking habit will be released. As your withdrawal symptoms disappear, it will become easier to concentrate and you will be more efficient at work and play. Your risk for heart attack and stroke will be reduced substantially. You will feel proud of your success and your newfound energy.

For each day you don't smoke, put the money you would have spent on cigarettes into a piggy bank. If you smoked a pack a day, in twenty years you will have increased your net worth by almost $20,000. That excludes any money you might have spent on medical bills to treat smoking-related illnesses.

If, by some miracle, all 30 million smokers in this country quit, our health care costs would be cut in half, doctors' offices would be much less crowded, and hospitals could be reduced to almost half their size.

The quit-smoking program described above works if you follow it faithfully. It did for me.

OTHER WAYS TO QUIT SMOKING

Surveys have shown that the vast majority of people who successfully quit smoking did so on their own. Despite that fact, smoking cessation has grown into a multimillion-dollar industry, especially in recent years as smoking bans in public places have spread like wildfire.

If you smoke, I hope you will not need to turn to the expensive smoking-cessation aids described below. The power to quit lies within you. You can use that power as you follow the program described above or something like it to wean yourself off cigarettes. The program I have set forth aims to help you fight withdrawal symptoms and keep you in control.

If you feel you need help, here are some of the aids available.

NICOTINE GUM. Nicotine replacement shows some promise of lessening withdrawal symptoms. The treatment comes in the form of chewing gum or a skin patch.

Nicorette, the nicotine gum, contains 2 to 4 milligrams of nicotine. Depending on how vigorously you chew, between 50 and 90 percent of the nicotine is released from the gum. Eighty percent is absorbed through the mucous membranes in your mouth. Coffee and carbonated beverages reduce the absorption rate.

A piece of gum should be chewed instead of lighting up anytime you feel a craving for a cigarette. Many people find the gum reduces their craving somewhat. The cost of Nicorette varies from pharmacy to pharmacy and, at this writing, is available only by prescription. One drugstore in central New Jersey sells the ninety-six-piece package for $33.45, while a nearby drugstore's price tag was $39. Nicorette's main side effect is that the gum may irritate the inside of the mouth.

NICOTINE PATCH. Unlike the gum, nicotine patches do not irritate the mouth or leave an unpleasant aftertaste, nor do they require incessant chewing. You wear the patch on the chest or arm for twenty-four hours before replacing it with a fresh patch.

A chemical on the patch opens the pores of the skin, allowing nicotine in the patch to slowly seep into the bloodstream. Once in the blood, the nicotine travels to the part of the brain where the cravings originate.

Several companies make nicotine patches, and the patches come in varying strengths and at varying prices. One Northeast pharmacy charged $43 for a box of fourteen patches containing 7 mg of nicotine each. The same brand with 21 mg of nicotine per patch cost $53. (A 14 mg patch also is available.) Your doctor can determine how strong a patch you need. Like the gum, nicotine patches are available by prescription only.

Nicotine patches have been proven effective in helping some people quit, but users are warned to smoke no cigarettes at all while wearing the patch. It's also important to refrain from smoking when chewing nicotine gum. Smoking while wearing the patch or chewing the gum effectively doubles the amount of nicotine being absorbed by your body. Absorbing so much nicotine at once causes a serious illness called nicotine poisoning. Nicotine poisoning can make the blood pressure fall, the heart race, and cause fainting.

CLONIDINE. Clonidine, a prescription medication developed to treat hypertension, has proved effective in relieving symptoms of opiate and alcohol withdrawal. Recently, it has been used successfully to ease nicotine withdrawal.

SMOKING-CESSATION CLINICS. Smoking-cessation clinics come in all sizes and shapes. Some are highly structured courses, professionally led by mental health professionals and costing several hundred dollars. Others are free self-help groups comprised of peers who meet in public libraries or community centers. Some workplaces have begun sponsoring quit-smoking classes for employees; often these classes are offered in conjunction with a new smoking ban. Many hospitals provide smoking-cessation courses on a sliding-scale fee. In some cases, you can get part of your enrollment fee refunded if you successfully finish the course.

Smoking-cessation classes that employ behavioral modification techniques have been shown to increase the effectiveness of the nicotine gum. Classes should be continued for several weeks after you have completely stopped smoking.

Regardless of how you try to quit smoking, try to remember that success generally comes after repeated failures. If you fall off the wagon and light up after not smoking for several days, don't construe it to mean you're incapable of quitting for good. Try again. It may be easier next time. And give yourself credit for trying. Be aware that smokers who try but fail to quit have a somewhat high incidence of depression. In these cases, your doctor may recommend an antidepressant medication.

Giving up smoking is difficult, perhaps one of the most difficult tasks you'll ever undertake. But the health benefits you will gain are far more significant than the temporary discomfort you'll experience during nicotine withdrawal.

CHAPTER 21

THE KRA DIET

Being overweight—as 30 percent of Americans are—forces the heart to work harder in order to pump blood through all that extra fatty tissue. Excess body fat also can contribute to hardening of the arteries, high blood pressure, and other problems. For some heart patients, losing weight can literally be a matter of life or death. With the average American diet deriving 50 percent of its calories from fat, it's no wonder that heart disease continues to be the leading killer in the United States.

The health perils, not to mention the cosmetic challenges, of being too fat are not lost on most Americans. Each year, we spend an estimated $2 billion on weight-loss diets. In 90 percent of cases where the dieter does lose weight, however, the lost pounds are regained in relatively short order.

Having treated thousands of overweight heart patients over the last two decades, I have heard countless complaints about how difficult it is to stick to a low-calorie, low-fat diet. To help my patients, I developed a diet plan that is easy to follow and extremely effective. The plan basically entails alternating between a fish day and a vegetable day Monday through Saturday, and rewarding yourself with a poultry or meat meal on Sunday. The Kra Diet includes ample helpings of pasta, breads, fruits, and grains, and certain oils, nuts, and other foods that have been scientifically shown to lower blood cholesterol. The diet also encourages a liberal use of spices to prevent your meals from becoming too bland.

If you are currently free of heart disease, following the Kra Diet will reduce your risk of developing heart problems in the future. If your coronary arteries are already narrowed, following my diet could reverse the disease process by reducing the amount of cholesterol plaque clogging your coronary arteries.

My diet achieves this goal by reducing your fat intake to approximately 10 percent, or less, of calories. You also will lower your daily cholesterol intake from the average 800 milligrams to less than 200 mg. By reducing dietary fat, the Kra Diet aims to lower your overall blood cholesterol level by 30 percent, your LDL level by at least 20 percent, and your triglyceride level by 30 to 40 percent. As explained in Chapter 3, LDL and triglycerides contribute to atherosclerosis.

WHY DIETS FAIL. Before reading the particulars of the Kra Diet, it helps to understand why so many diets fail. A major reason is that dieters often underestimate the number of calories they take in each day, according to a recent study in *The New England Journal of Medicine*. Counting calories is a mainstay of most diet programs, including mine. It therefore is crucial to keep an accurate daily log of how many calories you ingest in order to avoid this trap.

Another trap people fall into is conjuring up excuses

for gaining weight. My patients often attribute their weight gain to holidays, weddings, birthdays, cocktail parties, or business luncheons. Other patients cite unhappiness in their lives as a reason for gaining weight. For them, the only activity that seems to bring any pleasure is eating. Overeaters Anonymous, Weight Watchers, and other support groups have helped many people develop better eating habits.

Some patients complain that they hardly eat anything but cannot lose even a pound. Eating too little fools your body into thinking it is starving; the body's self-preservation response to calorie withdrawal is to slow down the metabolism. This means you are not burning as many calories as you normally would as you go about your normal activities.

Another reason people don't lose weight is because they fail to couple their diet with exercise. Even if you make no changes in your caloric intake, increasing your level of physical activity will enable you to burn more body fat than you are gaining (see Chapter 18).

HOW MANY CALORIES DO I NEED? To calculate your daily caloric requirement, multiply your ideal weight by 10. For example, a woman who should weigh 130 pounds needs at least 1,300 calories a day. In order to lose one pound, you must burn 3,500 to 4,000 calories. If you use up 1,500 calories a day with normal activity, and another 500 or so with exercise, while taking in only 1,500 calories, you will have a net loss of 500 calories a day. At the end of seven days, you will have lost 1 pound. In a month, you will have lost up to four to four and a half pounds. In one year, you theoretically could lose 52 pounds on the Kra Diet, although most people will shed a smaller but respectable 25 to 30 pounds.

KNOWING THE NUMBERS. As you embark on the Kra Diet, these basic facts should help you better track your calorie intake:

- One gram of fat contains nine calories. To find out how many calories of fat in the food you are about to eat, look at the label and multiply the number of grams of fat by nine.
- One gram of sugar contains four calories.

GETTING STARTED. Before you begin the diet, stock up on herbs and spices, such as basil, curry, chili powder, bay leaves, caraway seeds, cloves, ginger, garlic, mustard, nutmeg, oregano, peppercorns, sage, thyme, saffron, and any other spices you like. Spices greatly enhance the flavor of foods while adding no fat and very few calories to your meals.

Also buy some walnuts, a good source of Omega-3 fatty acid, the same that's in fish oil. Some of my physician friends munch on walnuts every day in order to lower their blood cholesterol and reduce their risk of heart attack.

WHAT TO EAT. Other items to buy for the Kra Diet are brown rice, black beans, low-fat yogurt, chickpeas, kidney beans, lentils, lima beans, great northern beans, and pinto beans. Also buy high-fiber foods, including oats, potatoes, barley, rice bran, wheat bran, graham crackers; and whole-grain breads such as rye and pumpernickel. Don't forget the fresh fruits and vegetables: apples, plums, peas, carrots, cabbage, broccoli, oranges, tangerines, and tomatoes, to name a few. Grains, fruit, and vegetables should be eaten every day. (Vegetable haters may enjoy low-salt vegetable juices, which are packed with nutrients.)

Pasta, another nutritious low-fat food, also can be eaten

daily. Eating pasta with garlic sautéed in olive oil is particularly good for your heart. The Italians eat plenty of it, and they boast the lowest heart-attack rate in Europe. Olive oil is high in monosaturated fat, which lowers blood cholesterol. Garlic also is getting a very good reputation for lowering the incidence of coronary artery disease. Studies expected to prove garlic's health benefits are under way in Germany.

Foods to eliminate from your diet include egg yolks and butter. Use cooking oils sparingly, except for olive oil, which should be included in as many meals as possible. Avoid coconut, palm, and other tropical oils because they are very high in saturated fats, which raise the blood cholesterol level. Food labels will tell you whether tropical oils are present.

Ideally, a vegetarian diet is best for the heart. But I have included in the Kra Diet fish, poultry, and small quantities of red meat to make it appealing to a wider audience. Most people find it difficult to maintain a strict vegetarian diet because they feel it diminishes their quality of life.

My simple "modified vegetarian" diet is designed to be followed six days a week. On the seventh day, you may reward yourself with your favorite meal. You may have a glass of wine each day with dinner or lunch.

As mentioned earlier, the Kra Diet alternates a total vegetarian day with a fish day. Chicken or beef days are sprinkled in once a week. Vegetables should be eaten every day, including the fish day and on the seventh "reward" day. Meat is permitted only once a week. Poultry cannot be used on the fish or vegetarian days. Three ounces of chicken without the skin has as much cholesterol (60 mg) as three ounces of beef. A serving should be no bigger than the palm of your hand.

The fish day need not be boring. Seafood is actually quite delicious if it's fresh and prepared properly. You may use shellfish anytime you like, but eat seafood either baked or broiled, not fried. Some people dislike seafood because of the smell and taste. Using lots of spices or baking fish in parchment paper masks the fishy taste. For example, you can brush scrod with olive, canola, or peanut oil, add some wine, garlic, and chives, and bake it in parchment paper or just broil it in the oven. You can use a small amount of a brown sauce to give your fish a little zest.

On vegetarian days, variety is key. You can stir-fry vegetables in a wok with spices and olive oil. You can steam vegetables and serve them over rice. You can add vegetables and legumes to soup, which is a nutritious addition to any meal. For example, lentil soup cooked with onions, tomatoes, carrots, and thyme is delicious. If you don't have time to cook soup from scratch, there is a growing variety of low-salt canned soups available.

On vegetarian days, you can whip up some pasta with tomato sauce or olive oil and garlic in minutes. Or use cholesterol-free eggs to make a vegetable omelet cooked in olive or safflower oil.

Breakfast is a natural with the Kra Diet. It can include whole grain cold cereals with skim milk, hot oatmeal, fruit juice, and toasted whole grain bread with jam.

GET ENOUGH FLUIDS. Be sure to drink two to three glasses of water in the morning and again in the afternoon. Keeping your fluid intake adequate promotes good kidney function and decreases your desire for food. Water retention can be negligible if you maintain a low-salt diet.

Try not to skip meals, especially breakfast, because it gives you energy and makes you less hungry for lunch.

The table at the end of this chapter provides calorie and cholesterol counts for common foods. Please consult your doctor before starting this diet.

SAMPLE MENUS

FISH DAY. Breakfast: Bran flakes; orange juice or a fruit; one slice of whole wheat, pumpernickel, or rye bread with low-fat cottage cheese, farmer cheese, low-fat American cheese, or goat cheese; a slice of tomato; coffee. Eating a low-fat bran muffin with jelly in lieu of the bread will further curb your lunchtime appetite.

Lunch: Tuna (water-packed) with onions, garlic, and tomatoes on a green salad; two water crackers. Tuna can be substituted with canned salmon, sardines, smoked trout, shrimp, scallops, oysters, or lobster salad with reduced-fat mayonnaise; low-fat yogurt for dessert.

Dinner: Any fish with spices, baked or broiled, served with brown rice and lima beans, or with dill sauce (made with grated onions, chopped dill, black pepper, lemon juice, and yogurt); salad of tomatoes with olive oil and vinegar, chives, garlic, and Dijon mustard; frozen low-fat yogurt, low-fat ice cream, or Italian ices for dessert; coffee or tea.

VEGETABLE DAY. Breakfast: Juice, bran flakes, banana, sliced dark bread with jelly, farmer or low-fat cottage cheese; coffee with low-fat milk.

Lunch: Large glass of salt-free vegetable juice, salad with olive oil, lentils, chives, and tomatoes; vegetable soup, crackers with tahini or hummus; unsalted air-popped popcorn.

Dinner: Lentil or minestrone soup; stir-fried vegetables of your choice or steamed vegetables with olive oil, garlic, pepper, and chives; brown rice or potatoes (not fried), or pasta with tomato sauce; two slices of dark bread; glass of wine; sherbet, Jell-O, or fruit for dessert.

SEVENTH DAY. On the seventh day, you may eat a lean steak, chicken, or veal, some cheese, or most anything else you crave. Be sure to include grains, such as bread, and complex carbohydrates, such as beans. Half an egg is permissible, but avoid butter and whole milk, and don't let your daily calorie count exceed 1,500.

At end of six weeks, the Kra Diet should reduce your overall blood cholesterol level to below 190, and your LDL to 130. If this has not happened, I recommend cholesterol-lowering medications if you have coronary artery disease or peripheral vascular disease (see Chapter 11).

This diet requires some imagination and creativity on your part. I have given you the outline; you must write the script. And, as with all diet programs, consult your doctor before embarking on it. People who have tried this diet enjoy the relative freedom it offers. Over the past ten years, I am pleased to report that it has worked wonders for many of my patients. I am hopeful it will do the same for you.

Glossary

Aerobics: Any form of sustained exercise that strengthens the heart and lungs; aerobic exercises include running, jogging, swimming, rowing, and bicycling.

Aneurysm: A weakened portion of a blood vessel that has ballooned out and is at risk of rupturing.

Angina: An attack of pain, tightness, or heaviness in the chest that can result when the heart muscle does not receive enough blood.

Angiography: A specialized X ray of the coronary arteries that is made after dye is injected into the bloodstream.

Angioplasty: See *balloon angioplasty*.

Angiotensin converting enzyme (ACE) inhibitors: A new class of medications used to treat high blood pressure and heart failure.

Antiarrhythmic: A type of medication used to treat irregular heartbeats.

Anticoagulant: Any drug that thins out the blood and prevents blood clots from forming.

Antihypertensive: Any drug designed to lower blood pressure.

Antioxidant: Any vitamin or medication that prevents a molecule from undergoing a chemical reaction called oxidation. Oxidation has been linked to heart disease and certain forms of cancer.

Aorta: The main artery of the body; originates from the left ventricle.

Aortic stenosis: A narrowing of the aortic valve of the heart.

Arteriogram: An X ray of arteries after a dye injection.

Arteriosclerosis: Thickened coronary arteries that have lost their normal elasticity as a result of the aging process; also known as hardening of the arteries.

Atherosclerosis: Hardened coronary arteries that have become narrowed or clogged with cholesterol plaques, fibrous tissue, and calcium; also known as coronary artery disease.

Atrial fibrillation: A condition in which the upper chambers of the heart contract at an irregular rate.

Atrium: Upper chamber of the heart.

Automatic implantable defibrillator: An implantable device that administers an electrical shock to normalize a dangerously fast heart rate.

Balloon angioplasty: A procedure in which a balloon is placed into a coronary artery via a catheter and inflated to flatten cholesterol plaques against the artery wall and restore adequate blood flow.

Beta-blocker: A class of medications used to treat angina, high blood pressure, and arrhythmias.

Beta-carotene: A provitamin of vitamin A.

Blood-thinner: A group of chemical substances that reduces the ability of the blood to clot (i.e. heparin, Coumadin).

Bradycardia: A heart rate below 60 beats per minute.

Calcium channel blockers: A group of medications that block the movement of calcium into certain cells of the body. Used to treat hypertension, angina, and irregular heart rhythms.

Cardiac arrest: Complete cessation of the heartbeat, which causes loss of consciousness because blood can no longer reach the brain.

Cardiac catheterization: The snaking of a long, flexible tube called a catheter from a blood vessel in the groin or arm into the chambers and arteries of the heart; used in diagnosis of coronary artery disease and disease of the heart valves.

Cardiomyopathy: Any form of heart muscle disease that reduces the heart's efficiency; caused by virus, metabolic reasons, and coronary artery disease.

Cardioversion: A treatment in which a patient is electrically shocked to revert an extremely fast regular or irregular heart rhythm to normal.

Carotid artery disease: A blockage in one or more of the four main arteries in the neck and head.

Cholesterol: A type of fat found in animal products. Cholesterol is necessary for cell metabolism and hormone production; excessive cholesterol in the blood has been shown to raise the risk of coronary artery disease.

Congestive heart failure (CHF): A condition in which fluid accumulates in the lungs, abdomen, and legs because the heart has lost its ability to pump blood efficiently.

Coronary artery: One of three main arteries that supply the heart muscle.

Coronary artery disease: A condition in which arteries supplying blood to the heart are narrowed or completely blocked by cholesterol plaques; also known as coronary heart disease.

Coronary bypass surgery: Surgery in which a blood vessel from the chest or leg is grafted onto a blocked coronary artery to create a bypass channel past the obstructed site.

Defibrillation: An electric shock administrated to a fibrillating (twitching) heart in order to restore a normal rhythm.

Diabetes: A metabolic disorder caused by a dearth of insulin-producing cells in the pancreas. Diabetics are unable to adequately metabolize dietary sugars, which results in too much glucose in the blood. Diabetics have an elevated risk for heart disease and other medical problems.

Diastolic blood pressure: The lower number of a blood pressure reading that corresponds to pressure inside the arteries during the relaxation phase of a heartbeat.

Digitalis: A medication derived from the foxglove plant used to treat heart failure and abnormal heart rhythms.

Digoxin: A medication similar to digitalis with the same uses.

Dissecting aneurysm: The tearing of the walls of an artery, allowing blood to leak between the layers of the arterial wall.

Echocardiogram: A sonar examination of the heart.

Eclampsia: Seizures and hypertension associated with pregnancy.

Electrocardiogram (ECG): A device that measures the electrical impulses of the heart.

Electrolytes: A variety of minerals and chemical compounds needed by all living cells. Carried by the blood, electrolytes include sodium, potassium, chloride, and carbon dioxide.

Electrophysiology: A new branch of cardiology that specializes in the diagnosis and treatment of irregular heart beats.

Embolism: A clot that travels from one site to another and blocks an artery.

Endarterectomy: A delicate and controversial operation to open blocked carotid arteries.

Endocarditis: Infection of the valves and linings of the heart.

Equilibrium radionuclide angiocardiogram: See *multigated graft acquisition test*.

Estrogen: A female hormone produced by the ovaries during the childbearing years. Estrogen-replacement therapy can be taken after menopause to lower the risk of heart disease and osteoporosis and to relieve menopausal symptoms.

Exercise stress test: A continuous electrocardiogram taken during exercise on a treadmill or stationary bicycle. The test is used to detect advanced coronary artery disease or to evaluate how much exercise a patient can do safely.

Extrasystoles: A skipped beat or extra heart beat.

Familial hypercholesterolemia: A genetic error affecting metabolism that produces high cholesterol that cannot be controlled through diet.

Heart attack: An event in which part of the heart muscle is damaged or destroyed as a result of blocked coronary arteries; also known as myocardial infarction.

Heart block: A condition in which the passage of impulses through the heart's conduction system is interrupted.

Heart failure: See *congestive heart failure*.

Heart murmur: A telltale sound made by the heart when one of its valves fails to open or close completely.

Heparin: A substance that prevents the clotting of blood.

High blood pressure: See *hypertension*.

High-density lipoprotein (HDL): A type of protein that carries cholesterol away from the coronary arteries; also known as "good cholesterol."

Hirudin: An anticoagulant derived from the leech.

Holter monitor: A portable electrocardiogram (ECG) that is worn for twenty-four to forty-eight hours.

Hypertension: High blood pressure.

Hypotension: Low blood pressure.

Ischemia: A condition in which the heart muscle becomes anemic due to a lack of oxygen, as in ischemic heart disease.

Labile hypertension: A condition in which blood pressure goes up and down throughout the day.

Libido: Sex drive.

Lipid profile: A blood test that measures the levels of LDL, HDL, and triglycerides.

Lipids: Cholesterol, triglycerides, and other fats.

Lipoprotein: Proteins that carry the lipids in the blood.

Low-density lipoprotein (LDL): A type of protein that carries cholesterol to the arteries, causing atherosclerosis; also known as "bad cholesterol."

Magnetic resonance imaging (MRI): A diagnostic machine that uses magnets and computers to create a three-dimensional image of internal organs.

Malignant hypertension: Extreme high blood pressure that comes on suddenly and requires emergency treatment.

Mitral valve prolapse syndrome: A condition in which one of the valves of the heart fails to close completely, allowing blood to leak between chambers; also known as floppy valve syndrome.

Monounsaturated fats: A family of fats, including olive oil, that help lower blood cholesterol.

Multigated graft acquisition test (MUGA): A sophisticated scan that uses radioactive dye, a gamma camera, and a computer to measure how well the heart is contracting and ejecting oxygenated blood; also known as an equilibrium radionuclide angiocardiogram.

Myocardial infarction: See *heart attack*.

Nitroglycerin: A drug that dilates arteries and used to treat angina.

Obesity: Being 20 to 30 percent over ideal weight.

Open-heart surgery: A heart operation during which the circulation is taken over by a heart-lung machine.

Orthostatic hypotension: A sudden drop in the blood pressure that can cause fainting.

Osteoporosis: A condition in which the bones lose so much calcium that they begin to break under the slightest pressure; primarily afflicts older women.

Pacemaker: A device placed in the heart to maintain an adequate heart rate.

Palpitations: A sensation that the heart is pounding too rapidly, irregularly, or too strongly.

Paroxysmal tachycardia: A condition in which the heart rate accelerates to 130 to 260 beats per minute.

Percutaneous transluminal coronary angioplasty (PTCA): Using a balloon catheter to open a blocked artery; also known as balloon angioplasty.

Pericarditis: An inflammation of the membrane that covers the heart.

Peripheral vascular disease (PVD): A narrowing of arteries in the neck, arms, and legs usually caused by cholesterol plaques.

Persantine thallium stress test: A modified stress test performed on people with orthopedic problems or who otherwise cannot undergo a regular thallium exercise stress test.

Phlebitis: An inflammation of the veins in the arms or legs.

Plaque: Fatty deposits in the arteries that constrict blood flow, causing atherosclerosis.

Pneumothorax: A collapsed lung.

Polyunsaturated fats: A family of animal or vegetable fats, including canola, corn, safflower, and sunflower oils; may help lower blood cholesterol levels.

Progesterone: A female hormone that may be given in conjunction with estrogen-replacement therapy in order to reduce the risk of uterine cancer.

Pulmonary embolism: A potentially fatal condition in which a blood clot travels to the pulmonary artery.

Restenosis: A reblock of a coronary artery that had been previously opened with balloon angioplasty.

Saturated fats: A family of fats, such as beef fat, palm, coconut, and other tropical oils, that have been implicated in raising the blood cholesterol level.

Sclerotherapy: Injections of a special solution into varicose veins in order to collapse them.

Splenic flexure: A bend in the left part of small intestine adjacent to the heart; gas is commonly trapped there, causing chest pain that can be mistaken for a heart attack.

Stenosis: A narrowing and obstruction of an artery.

Superficial phlebitis: The appearance of varicose veins near the surface of the skin.

Supraventricular tachycardia: A very rapid, regular heartbeat.

Syndrome X: A diagnosis given to someone who suffers chest pain but has no evidence of coronary artery disease.

Systolic blood pressure: The upper number of a blood pressure that corresponds to the pressure against the arteries during a contraction of the heart.

Tachycardia: When the resting heart rate accelerates to more than one hundred beats per minute.

Thallium stress test: An exercise stress test involving the injection of radioactive thallium into the bloodstream during exercise. The heart is scanned by a gamma camera, allowing doctors to visualize flow of blood through the coronary arteries. If there is a blockage, the thallium cannot enter the heart.

Thrombolysis: Drug therapy to dissolve a blood clot that has caused a heart attack.

Thrombophlebitis: A combination of blood clots and inflammation in a vein.

Thrombosis: A blood clot.

Transient ischemic attack (TIA): Temporary symptoms of a stroke caused by the disruption of blood to the brain. This can be the forerunner of a full blown stroke.

Triglycerides: A lipid (fat) found in the blood and fatty tissue of the body (i.e. adipose tissue of the belly).

Vago-vagal attack: A reflex nervous response to an unpleasant situation or to pain; most common cause of temporary drop in blood pressure.

Varicose veins: Swollen blood vessels that result when valves in the leg veins are faulty, allowing blood to pool.

Ventricle: Lower chamber of the heart.

Ventricular tachycardia: An abnormally rapid heart rhythm that can lead to sudden death.

Tables

Salt (Sodium) and Calorie Content of Common Foods*

Food Item	Common Measure (Weight, g)	Sodium, mg	Calories
	Beverages (Alcoholic)		
Beer, regular	12-oz can or bottle (360)	18	151
Beer, light	12-oz can or bottle (360)	14	70–136
Brandy	1½ fl oz (45)	1	105
Gin (86 proof)	1½ fl oz (45)	1	105
Rum (86 proof)	1½ fl oz (45)	1	105
Vodka (86 proof)	1½ fl oz (45)	Trace	105
Whiskey, bourbon, rye, or scotch (86 proof)	1½ fl oz (45)	1	105
Wine, red domestic	4 fl oz (120)	12	99
Wine, red imported	4 fl oz (120)	6	99
Wine, sherry	4 fl oz (120)	14	161
Wine, white domestic	4 fl oz (120)	19	99
Wine, white imported	4 fl oz (120)	2	99

*Source USDA

Food Item	Common Measure (Weight, g)	Sodium, mg	Calories
Beverages (Nonalcoholic)			
Apple juice	6 fl oz (180)	4	87
Coffee, brewed	1 cup—8 fl oz (240)	2	0
Coffee, instant	1 cup—8 fl oz (240)	1	2
Cranberry juice cocktail	6 fl oz (180)	3	123
Grape juice, bottled or canned	6 fl oz (190)	6	125
Orange juice, fresh	6 fl oz (180)	4	84
Orange juice, frozen	6 fl oz (186)	4	92
Pineapple juice	6 fl oz (188)	3	69
Prune juice	6 fl oz (192)	4	149
Soft drink			
Regular	8 fl oz (240)	11	96
Diet	8 fl oz (240)	29	1
Club soda	8 fl oz (240)	56	0
Collins mix	8 fl oz (240)	20	112
Quinine water (tonic)	8 fl oz (240)	2	72
Mineral water	8 fl oz (240)	42	0
Tea	1 cup—8 fl oz (240)	1	0
Tea, instant	1 cup—8 fl oz (240)	2	0
Tomato juice	6 fl oz (192)	659	36
Vegetable juice cocktail	6 fl oz (182)	665	30
Breads and Crackers			
Biscuit, home recipe	1 biscuit (28)	175	103
Biscuit, mix, with milk	1 biscuit (28)	272	104
Bread, French	1 slice (23)	116	64
Bread, pumpernickel	1 slice (32)	182	79
Bread, rye	1 slice (25)	139	61
Bread, white	1 slice (25)	114	76
Bread, whole wheat	1 slice (25)	132	61
Bread stick, salt coating	1 stick, small (10)	167	38
Bread stick, without salt coating	1 stick, small (10)	70	38

Food Item	Common Measure (Weight, g)	Sodium, mg	Calories
Breads and Crackers (cont.)			
Cracker, saltine or soda	1 cracker (3)	35	12
Cracker, soup or oyster	10 crackers (8)	83	33
Roll, dinner, brown and serve	1 roll (28)	138	83
Roll, frankfurter, hamburger	1 roll (40)	202	119
Roll, hard	1 roll (50)	313	156
Cereals (Non-Sugar-Coated)			
Bran, all	1 oz—⅓ cup (28)	160	70
Bran flakes (40%)	1 oz—⅔ cup (28)	265	90
Corn Chex	1 oz—1 cup (28)	325	110
Corn flakes	1 oz—1 cup (28)	350	110
Granola	1 oz—¼ cup (28)	75	130
Grits, cooked	1 oz—¾ cup (28)	10	100
Oat flakes	1 oz—⅔ cup (28)	275	100
Oatmeal, regular, without salt	1 oz—⅓ cup (28)	1	109
Oatmeal, instant, regular flavor (salt added)	1 oz—¾ cup (28)	252	105
Rice, cream of, unsalted	1 oz—¾ cup (28)	10	110
Rice, puffed	½ oz—1 heaping cup (14)	10	50
Rice Chex	1 oz—1⅛ cup (28)	275	110
Rice Crispies	1 oz—1 cup (28)	340	110
Wheat Chex	1 oz—⅔ cup (28)	240	110
Wheat, cream of, regular	1 oz—¾ cup (28)	7	110
Wheat flakes	1 oz—1 cup (28)	370	110
Wheat, puffed	½ oz—1 heaping cup (14)	10	50
Wheat, shredded	1 large biscuit (21)	1	80
Condiments, Dressings, and Seasonings			
Barbecue sauce	1 tbsp (16)	130	14
Chili sauce	1 tbsp (17)	227	16
Ketchup, tomato	1 tbsp (15)	156	16
Mayonnaise	1 tbsp (15)	78	101

Food Item	Common Measure (Weight, g)	Sodium, mg	Calories
Condiments, Dressings, and Seasonings (cont.)			
Mustard, prepared	1 tsp (5)	65	5
Parsley flakes	1 tbsp (4)	2	2
Pepper, black	1 tsp (2)	1	8
Salad dressings			
Blue cheese or Roquefort	1 tbsp (15)	153	76
French	1 tbsp (14)	214	66
Italian	1 tbsp (15)	116	83
Russian	1 tbsp (15)	133	74
Thousand Island	1 tbsp (16)	109	80
Oil and vinegar	1 tbsp (15)	Trace	62
Salt, table	1 tsp (6)	2,325	0
Soy sauce	1 tbsp (18)	1,029	12
Sugar, granulated	1 tsp (4)	Trace	15
Worcestershire sauce	1 tbsp (17)	206	Trace
Dairy Products, Eggs, and Margarine			
Butter, regular	1 tbsp (14)	116	102
Butter, unsalted, regular	1 tbsp (14)	2	102
Butter, whipped	1 tbsp (9)	74	69
Cheese, American	1 slice—1 oz (28)	406	116
Cheese, cheddar	1 oz (28)	176	114
Cheese, cottage	½ cup (113)	457	117
Cheese, cream	1 oz (28)	84	99
Cheese, Parmesan, grated	1 oz (28)	528	129
Cheese, processed spread	1 oz (28)	381	82
Cheese, Swiss	1 oz (28)	74	107
Cream, half and half	1 tbsp (15)	7	20
Cream, heavy	1 tbsp (15)	6	53
Cream, sour	1 tbsp (12)	6	26
Egg, whole	1 medium (50)	69	79
Egg, white	1 medium (33)	50	16
Egg, yolk	1 medium (17)	8	63
Margarine, regular	1 tbsp (14)	133	100
Margarine, soft, tub	1 tbsp (14)	152	100
Margarine, unsalted	1 tbsp (14)	1	100
Milk, buttermilk	8 fl oz (245)	257	99
Milk, low-fat (2%)	8 fl oz (244)	122	121

Food Item	Common Measure (Weight, g)	Sodium, mg	Calories
Dairy Products, Eggs, and Margarine (cont.)			
Milk, skim	8 fl oz (245)	126	86
Milk, whole	8 fl oz (244)	120	150
Desserts			
Brownies	1 average (20)	50	97
Cake, angel food	1 slice, 1/12 cake (56)	134	150
Cake, devil's food, chocolate icing	1 slice, 1/12 cake (67)	120	260
Cake, pound	1 medium slice (55)	171	225
Cake, white, white icing	1 slice 1/12 cake (104)	243	290
Cake, yellow, with caramel icing	1 slice, 1/12 cake (108)	79	391
Cookies, chocolate chip	1 cookie, medium (11)	35	50
Cookies, fig	1 bar (14)	48	56
Cookies, oatmeal	1 cookie (13)	27	120
Cookies, sandwich	1 cookie (10)	40	63
Cookies, shortbread	1 cookie (8)	29	37
Cookies, sugar	1 cookie (26)	108	128
Cookies, vanilla wafer	1 wafer (4)	9	16
Gelatin, plain	½ cup (120)	60	80
Ice cream	1 cup (140)	112	257
Ice milk	1 cup (131)	105	199
Pie, apple	1 slice, ⅛ pie (71)	208	182
Pie, banana cream	1 slice, ⅙ pie (66)	90	128
Pie, blueberry	1 slice, ⅛ pie (71)	163	172
Pie, cherry	1 slice, ⅛ pie (71)	169	185
Pie, chocolate cream	1 slice, ⅙ pie (66)	80	174
Pie, lemon meringue	1 slice, ⅛ pie (105)	296	268
Pie, mince	1 slice, ⅛ pie (71)	241	259
Pie, peach	1 slice, ⅛ pie (71)	169	150
Pie, pecan	1 slice, ⅛ pie (71)	241	259
Pie, pumpkin	1 slice, ⅛ pie (71)	169	150
Pudding, bread	½ cup (133)	267	248
Pudding, chocolate, home recipe	½ cup (130)	73	198
Pudding, chocolate, mix	½ cup (148)	195	322

FOOD ITEM	COMMON MEASURE (WEIGHT, G)	SODIUM, MG	CALORIES
	Desserts (cont.)		
Pudding, rice	½ cup (132)	94	194
Pudding, tapioca	½ cup (83)	129	111
Pudding, vanilla, home recipe	½ cup (128)	83	142
Pudding, vanilla, mix	½ cup (148)	200	321
Sherbet, orange	1 cup (193)	89	259
	Fish and Seafood		
Bluefish, broiled or baked with butter	4 oz (114)	117	219
Clams, raw	4 to 5—3 oz (85)	174	56
Cod, broiled with butter	4 oz (114)	125	99
Crabmeat, canned, drained	1 can—4 oz (114)	1,250	126
Flounder, baked with butter	4 oz (114)	268	102
Haddock, fried	4 oz (114)	200	162
Halibut, broiled with butter	4 oz (114)	152	191
Lobster, boiled, meat only	4 oz (114)	183	123
Oysters, fresh	6 small—2 oz (58)	75	38
Salmon, broiled or baked with butter	4 oz (114)	133	207
Sardines, drained	1 can—3¼ oz (92)	598	187
Scallops, bay, steamed	10 to 12—4 oz (114)	302	153
Shrimp, raw	10 jumbo—3 oz (85)	137	98
Tuna, chunk, canned in oil, drained	1 can—3¼ oz (92)	328	182
Tuna, chunk, canned in water, drained	1 can—3¼ oz (92)	312	117
	Fruits		
Apple	1 medium (138)	2	118
Applesauce, sweetened	½ cup (125)	3	227

Food Item	Common Measure (Weight, g)	Sodium, mg	Calories
	Fruits (cont.)		
Apricots, canned, syrup	½ cup (129)	13	111
Apricots, dried	5 halves, medium (24)	2	62
Banana	1 medium (119)	2	68
Blackberries	½ cup (72)	1	42
Blueberries	½ cup (72)	1	45
Cantaloupe	½ melon (272)	24	47
Cherries, sweet, whole	1 cup (130)	2	82
Cherries, canned	1 cup (257)	10	110
Fruit cocktail, canned in syrup	1 cup (255)	15	195
Fruit cocktail, canned in water	1 cup (255)	15	95
Grapefruit	½ grapefruit (120)	1	26
Grapefruit, canned	½ cup (127)	2	89
Grapes	10 grapes (50)	1	23
Honeydew	⅕ melon (298)	28	61
Orange	1 medium (131)	1	47
Peach, skinned	1 medium (100)	1	29
Peaches, canned, syrup	½ cup (128)	8	100
Peaches, canned, water	½ cup (128)	8	38
Pear	1 medium (168)	1	93
Pears, canned, syrup	½ cup (128)	8	98
Pears, canned, water	½ cup (128)	8	40
Pineapple, fresh	1 cup (135)	1	71
Pineapple, canned, syrup	1 cup (255)	4	189
Pineapple, canned, water	1 cup (246)	4	96
Plums	10 plums (66)	1	30
Plums, canned, water	1 cup (256)	10	111
Prunes, cooked	½ cup (107)	4	108
Prunes, dried	5 prunes (43)	2	95
Raisins	¼ cup, packed (36)	4	98
Rhubarb, cooked, sweetened	½ cup (135)	3	190
Strawberries	½ cup (75)	1	28
Strawberries, frozen, sweetened	½ cup (128)	1	139
Watermelon	1/16 melon (426)	8	55

Food Item	Common Measure (Weight, g)	Sodium, mg	Calories
	Meat and Poultry		
Bacon, regular	2 slices—½ oz (14)	274	61
Bacon, Canadian	1 slice—1 oz (28)	394	58
Beef, corned	2 slices—3 oz (85)	802	315
Beef, fried, creamed	1 cup (245)	1,754	377
Beef, ground, lean	1 patty—4 oz (114)	76	249
Beef, lean, rump roast	2 slices—4 oz (114)	74	237
Beef, lean, round steak	6 oz (170)	180	444
Bologna	1 slice (22)	224	61
Chicken, broiler	¼ chicken (147)	58	120
Chicken, fried	1 drumstick (56)	49	88
Chicken, roasted	½ breast (98)	69	99
Frankfurter, all meat	1 frankfurter (57)	639	176
Ham, cured lean	2 slices—4 oz (114)	1,494	330
Ham, cured, country, lean	2 slices—4 oz (144)	980	304
Ham, fresh, lean	2 slices—4 oz (114)	79	426
Ham, chopped, lunchmeat	1 slice (21)	288	62
Ham, deviled	1 oz (28)	253	100
Lamb, loin chop, lean	2 chops—4 oz (114)	79	214
Lamb, leg, lean	2 slices—4 oz (114)	78	212
Liver, calf, fried	3 slices—4 oz (114)	133	298
Liver, chicken, simmered	5 livers—4 oz (114)	56	188
Liverwurst (braunschweiger)	1 slice (28)	324	88
Pork, loin roast, lean	1 slice—4 oz (114)	93	292
Salami, cooked, beef and pork	1 slice (22)	255	88
Salami, dry, beef and pork	1 slice (10)	226	45
Sausage, pork	1 link (13)	168	65

Food Item	Common Measure (Weight, g)	Sodium, mg	Calories
	Meat and Poultry (cont.)		
Sausage, pork	1 patty—2 oz (57)	259	129
Thuringer (summer sausage)	1 slice (22)	320	68
Turkey, dark meat	3 slices—4 oz (114)	91	218
Turkey, light meat	3 slices—4 oz (114)	61	200
Turkey, roll	1 oz (28)	166	70
Veal, cutlet, loin	1 cutlet—4 oz (114)	93	267
	Pasta		
Macaroni, plain, cooked	1 cup (140)	2	155
Macaroni with cheese	1 cup (200)	1,086	430
Pizza with cheese	1 slice—2 oz (57)	380	147
Pizza with sausage	1 slice—2 oz (57)	335	157
Spaghetti, with tomato sauce and cheese	1 cup (250)	955	190
Spaghetti, with tomato sauce, meatballs, and cheese	1 cup (248)	1,009	332
Soups, Commercial Varieties, Condensed (Prepared with Addition of Equal Volumes of Water, Unless Noted)			
Bean	1 cup (250)	1,008	168
Beef broth	1 cup (241)	1,152	64
Chicken, cream of (with milk)	1 cup (245)	1,054	179
Chicken noodle	1 cup (240)	1,107	62
Chicken with rice	1 cup (241)	814	48
Clam chowder, Manhattan	1 cup (244)	938	81
Clam chowder, New England (with milk)	1 cup (248)	992	139
Minestrone	1 cup (241)	911	105
Mushroom, cream of (with milk)	1 cup (248)	992	216
Onion	1 cup (240)	1,051	65

Food Item	Common Measure (Weight, g)	Sodium, mg	Calories
Soups (cont.)			
Pea, green	1 cup (250)	987	130
Tomato	1 cup (245)	872	88
Tomato, cream of (with milk)	1 cup (250)	932	173
Turkey noodle	1 cup (240)	998	79
Vegetable beef	1 cup (245)	957	78
Vegetarian vegetable	1 cup (245)	823	78
Vegetables (Considered Fresh, Unless Listed Otherwise; Considered Cooked, Unless Indicated as Raw. Sodium Content of Cooked Vegetables Is Content Before Salt Is Added.)			
Artichoke	1 bud (120)	36	12
Asparagus	4 spears (60)	4	12
Asparagus, canned	4 spears (80)	298	17
Beans, baked, canned, with pork and tomato sauce	½ cup (145)	464	156
Beans, baked, canned, with pork and molasses sauce	½ cup (145)	303	192
Beans, green	½ cup (63)	3	16
Beans, green, canned	½ cup (65)	319	16
Beans, green, frozen	½ cup (68)	1	17
Beans, lima	½ cup (85)	1	95
Beans, lima, canned	½ cup (85)	228	82
Beans, lima, frozen	½ cup (85)	64	84
Beets	½ cup (85)	37	27
Beets, canned	½ cup (85)	240	42
Broccoli	1 stalk, medium (151)	18	39
Broccoli, frozen	½ cup (94)	18	24
Brussels sprouts	4 sprouts (84)	8	30
Brussels sprouts, frozen	½ cup (77)	8	26
Cabbage	½ cup (72)	8	16
Cabbage, raw	½ cup (35)	4	11
Carrots	½ cup (78)	26	34
Carrots, frozen	½ cup (113)	52	35

Food Item	Common Measure (Weight, g)	Sodium, mg	Calories
	Vegetables (cont.)		
Carrots, raw	1 medium (72)	34	12
Cauliflower	½ cup (63)	6	14
Cauliflower, frozen	½ cup (90)	9	16
Cauliflower, raw	½ cup (58)	8	14
Celery, raw	1 stalk (20)	25	7
Corn	1 ear (140)	1	70
Corn, canned, creamed	½ cup (128)	336	105
Corn, canned, whole kernel	½ cup (83)	192	87
Cucumber, raw	6 large slices (28)	2	4
Lettuce, head, raw	¼ head (135)	12	18
Lettuce, leaf, raw	1 cup (55)	5	10
Mushrooms	½ cup (35)	4	10
Okra	5 pods (53)	1	16
Onions, green, raw, with tops	2 medium (30)	2	14
Onions, raw	1 tbsp (10)	1	4
Peas, green	½ cup (80)	1	57
Peas, green, canned	½ cup (85)	247	82
Peas, green, frozen	½ cup (85)	106	55
Peppers, sweet	½ cup (75)	13	22
Pickles, dill	1 spear (30)	232	3
Pickles, sweet gherkin	1 whole pickle (15)	128	22
Potato, baked or boiled	1 medium (156)	5	145
Potatoes, french-fried, unsalted	10 strips (50)	15	137
Potatoes, mashed, milk and salt added	1 cup (210)	632	137
Radishes, raw	5 medium (18)	8	7
Sauerkraut	½ cup (235)	777	21
Spinach, canned	½ cup (103)	455	25
Spinach, frozen	½ cup (50)	78	24
Spinach, raw	½ cup (55)	25	7
Squash, summer	½ cup (105)	3	13
Sweet potato, boiled	1 medium (132)	20	126
Sweet potato, canned	1 medium (100)	48	107

Food Item	Common Measure (Weight, g)	Sodium, mg	Calories
Vegetables (cont.)			
Tomato, raw	1 medium (123)	14	27
Tomatoes, canned	½ cup (120)	195	26
Snacks			
Candy, milk chocolate	1 oz (28)	28	147
Caramels, plain or chocolate	1 oz (28)	74	113
Corn chips, regular	1 oz (28)	231	157
Doughnuts, cake type, plain	1 doughnut (32)	160	125
Mints, chocolate-coated	1 small (11)	20	45
Nuts, cashews, dry-roasted, salted	4 tbsp—1 oz (28)	150	159
Peanut butter	1 tbsp—1 oz (16)	81	94
Peanuts, dry-roasted, salted	4 tbsp—1 oz (28)	123	166
Peanuts, roasted in oil, unsalted	4 tbsp—1 oz (28)	1	208
Popcorn, salted with butter	1 cup (9)	175	41
Popcorn, unsalted	1 cup (6)	1	23
Potato chips	14 chips—1 oz (28)	285	161
Pretzels, regular twist	5 pretzels—½ oz (14)	505	117

Cholesterol Content of Common Foods*

FOOD	AMOUNT	CHOLESTEROL (IN MILLIGRAMS)
	Meat Group	
	RED MEATS	
Bacon	2 slices	15
Beef (lean)	3 ounces	77
Frankfurter	2 (4 ounces)	112
Ham, boiled	2 ounces	51
Kidney, beef	3 ounces	315
Lamb (lean)	3 ounces	85
Liver, beef	3 ounces	372
Pork (lean)	3 ounces	75
Veal (lean)	3 ounces	84
	FOWL	
Chicken (dark meat, no skin)	3 ounces	77
Chicken (light meat, no skin)	3 ounces	65
Eggs (whole or yolk only)	1 large	252
Turkey (dark meat, no skin)	3 ounces	86
Turkey (white meat, no skin)	3 ounces	65
	FISH	
Clams, raw	3 ounces	43
Crab, canned	3 ounces	85
Flounder	3 ounces	69
Haddock	3 ounces	42
Halibut	3 ounces	50
Lobster	3 ounces	71
Mackerel	3 ounces	84
Oysters, raw	3 ounces	42
Salmon, canned	3 ounces	30
Sardines	3 ounces	119
Scallops	3 ounces	45
Shrimp, canned	3 ounces	128
Tuna, canned	3 ounces	55

*Source: USDA

Food	Amount	Cholesterol (in milligrams)
	Milk Group	
Butter	1 tablespoon	35
Buttermilk	1 cup	5
Cheese, cottage (4% fat)	½ cup	24
Cheese, cottage (1% fat)	½ cup	12
Cheese, cream	1 ounce	31
Cheese, hard	1 ounce	24–28
Cheese, spread	1 ounce	18
Chocolate milk (low-fat)	1 cup	20
Cream, heavy	1 tablespoon	21
Ice cream	½ cup	27
Ice milk	½ cup	13
Milk, skim	1 cup	5
Milk (1% fat)	1 cup	14
Milk (2% fat)	1 cup	22
Milk, whole	1 cup	34
Yogurt (low-fat)	1 cup	17
	Bread Group	
Angel food cake	1 slice	0
Chocolate cupcake	2½ inch diameter	17
Cornbread	1 ounce	58
Lemon meringue pie	⅛ of 9-inch pie	98
Muffin, plain	3-inch diameter	21
Noodles, egg	1 cup	50
Pancakes	7 tablespoons batter	54
Sponge cake	1/12 of 10-inch cake	162

Index

Index

Index

Index